Praise

"*The Modern Trauma Toolkit* is a comprehensive collection of exercises that will enable the reader to experience the often-forgotten universal wisdom that healing is dependent on feeling safe enough to invite our nervous system to be a collaborator on our personal journey to health."

—Stephen W. Porges, PhD, author of *Polyvagal Safety: Attachment, Communication, Self-Regulation* and *The Polyvagal Theory: Neurophysiological Foundations of Emotions, Attachment, Communication, and Self-regulation*; Founding Director, Traumatic Stress Research Consortium, Kinsey Institute, Indiana University Bloomington; Professor of Psychiatry, University of North Carolina at Chapel Hill

"Dr. Gibson's gem of a book is a succinct and penetrating primer on trauma and approaches to its treatment. Easy to read without being simplistic, it is a welcome introduction to this endemic phenomenon that affects us all both on the social and personal levels."

—Dr. Gabor Maté, MD, Family Medicine Physician, author of *The Myth of Normal: Trauma, Illness, and Healing in a Toxic Culture* and *In the Realm of Hungry Ghosts: Close Encounters with Addiction*

"*The Modern Trauma Toolkit* is the most compassionate, welcoming, and practical book on trauma recovery that I have seen. It is now my first recommendation to many who have suffered trauma."
—Jeffrey Rediger, MD, MDiv, Psychiatrist Physician, Faculty of Harvard Medical School, Medical Director of McLean SE Adult Psychiatry Community Affairs at McLean Hospital, and Chief of Behavioral Medicine at Good Samaritan Medical Center, author of *Cured: The Life-Changing Science of Spontaneous Healing*

"What a blessing that *The Modern Trauma Toolkit* is finally here! Christy Gibson shows up like a trusted friend, with a book that democratizes healing, a social justice–conscious book for the people, for *all* people, who have been hurt and yearn to both understand and apply self-help tools for safe, grounded nervous system healing. This is the book for anyone who is committed to the healing path—focusing on resilience, self-compassion, and what is good and right within us all."
—Lissa Rankin MD, Ob-Gyn Physician, author of *Mind Over Medicine: Scientific Proof That You Can Heal Yourself* and *Sacred Medicine: A Doctor's Quest to Unravel the Mysteries of Healing*

"Dr. Christy Gibson's compassionate, wise voice is one you want whispering in your ear as you work toward the life you deserve. Accessible, actionable, inclusive, comforting, and hopeful. A practical, inspired, and deeply intuitive contribution to a critical field."
—Jillian Horton, MD, Internal Medicine Physician; Associate Chair of the Department of Internal Medicine and Director at the Alan Klass Medical Humanities Program at the Max Rady College of Medicine in Winnipeg, Manitoba; author of *We Are All Perfectly Fine: A Memoir of Love, Medicine, and Healing*

"In *The Modern Trauma Toolkit*, Dr. Christine Gibson invites the reader into a courageous exploration of what it means to be human, to survive painful things, as well as the impact of collective trauma. She teaches easily accessible and powerful healing tools that galvanize the journey toward post-traumatic growth. Her presence and care are tangible within each page of the book. Every step of the way, one can feel her presence as both a loving, wise guide and a compassionate, supportive cheerleader. This beautifully written book is sure to become a staple for healing practitioners and survivors alike."

—Kate Truitt, PhD, MBA, CEO of the Trauma Counseling Center of Los Angeles, Founder of the Amy Research Foundation, Developer of the Havening Techniques, author of *Healing In Your Hands: Self-Havening Practices to Harness Neuroplasticity, Heal Traumatic Stress, and Build Resilience*

"Trauma is a root cause of so much poor health across age groups and demographics. In her book *The Modern Trauma Toolkit* Dr. Gibson makes what we know about trauma, its impacts and how to address it accessible for everyone. This book is a must-read for clinicians and individuals looking for individualized tools to help them process their own experiences in a safe and approachable way."

—Katharine Smart, MD, Pediatric Emergency Medicine Physician Past President of Canadian Medical Association

"*The Modern Trauma Toolkit* is easily one of the most readable and balanced trauma books on the market. It's equipped with psychoeducation, case studies, and coping tools within the chapters to allow readers to not only make sense of some of the symptoms they may be experiencing but also practice coping. This is one of few trauma books that is culturally responsive, trauma informed, and inclusive of many different identities and experiences. An effortless read—educational, yet practical, you'll be glad you picked this up."

—Simone Saunders BSW, MSW, RSW, Managing Director of The Cognitive Corner

"*The Modern Trauma Toolkit* is by far the most well-organized, socially conscious, approachable, and actionable book on trauma healing I've ever read. Dr. Gibson is a brilliant and humble guide taking you through the process of rewiring your brain for wellness. Run, don't walk, to buy this book for you and anyone you know who wants to get back into the driver's seat of their life."

—Jen Wolkin, PhD, Neuropsychologist, author of
Quick Calm: Easy Meditations to Short-Circuit
Stress Using Mindfulness and Neuroscience

"Dr. Gibson's [book] is a down-to-earth collection of easy-to-read information for anyone who wants to understand more about trauma's impact on the mind and body—along with practical approaches for healing outside of traditional medical settings. There is something for everyone here from seasoned medical professionals who want to further support their patients with a trauma-informed approach and everyday community members just beginning their healing journey."

—Logan Cohen, Licensed Marriage and
Family Therapist, author of
How To (Hu)Man Up In Modern Society:
Heal Yourself and Save the World

"This book has been worth the wait! *The Modern Trauma Toolkit* by Dr Gibson is full of practical tools and exercises to help individuals at any stage of their healing journey. This is also a great guide for therapists looking to hone their skills and add some more resources to their clinical toolbox."

—Patrice Berry, PhD, Licensed Psychologist,
author of *Turning Crisis into Clarity:*
How to Survive or Thrive in the
Midst of Uncertainty

"The Modern Trauma Toolkit takes complex trauma theories and psychoeducation and breaks them into digestible information for any reader. The author does a fantastic job of personalizing the advice and invites the reader to explore their needs in a trauma-informed, gentle way. This book provides invaluable skills and body-based resources that will benefit all readers."

—Lauren Rasmussen, Certified Trauma Informed Coach and NARM Practitioner, Founder of The Simplest Self Wellness Inc.

"The Modern Trauma Toolkit is a gem. As a practicing psychologist and trauma therapist, I've read many trauma books over the years. Few are as accessible, personalized, body based, science backed, and resonant as this one. Dr. Gibson combines her professional and personal experiences into a highly readable and skimmable text, full of examples, exercises, anecdotes, explanatory graphics, and in-the-moment practices. Most trauma books are not written in a way that is actually trauma informed. It is clear that Dr. Gibson had her audience in mind when writing."

—Dr. Han Ren, Ph.D. Licensed Psychologist, Speaker, Educator

"The Modern Trauma Toolkit is an asset for anyone on the journey of healing from trauma. Dr. Gibson explains what happens in trauma and provides the latest therapeutic approaches, with time-honoured traditions, in a way that is accessible to all. With examples and exercises, readers can test out simple practices that can help bring them back to a calm state. It will surely help those living with trauma navigate the path to their post-traumatic growth."

—Dr. Shailla Vaidya, MD, Family and Emergency Medicine, Mind-Body Practitioner

THE MODERN TRAUMA TOOLKIT

NURTURE YOUR POST-TRAUMATIC GROWTH
WITH PERSONALIZED SOLUTIONS

Christy Gibson, MD

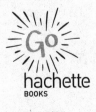

hachette
BOOKS

NEW YORK

Copyright © 2023 by Christine Gibson

Cover design by Sara Pinsonault
Cover copyright © 2023 by Hachette Book Group, Inc.

Hachette Go, an imprint of Hachette Books
Hachette Book Group
1290 Avenue of the Americas
New York, NY 10104
HachetteGo.com
Facebook.com/HachetteGo
Instagram.com/HachetteGo

First Edition: May 2023

Hachette Books is a division of Hachette Book Group, Inc.

The Hachette Go and Hachette Books name and logos are trademarks of Hachette Book Group, Inc.

The Hachette Speakers Bureau provides a wide range of authors for speaking events. To find out more, go to hachettespeakersbureau.com or email HachetteSpeakers@hbgusa.com.

Hachette Go books may be purchased in bulk for business, educational, or promotional use. For information, please contact your local bookseller or Hachette Book Group Special Markets Department at special.markets@hbgusa.com.

The publisher is not responsible for websites (or their content) that are not owned by the publisher.

Library of Congress Cataloging-in-Publication Data has been applied for.

ISBNs: 978-0-306-83106-5 (trade paperback); 978-0-306-83107-2 (ebook)

Printed in the United States of America

LSC-C

Printing 1, 2023

Contents

SOMATICS

SYSTEM SOLUTIONS

EXTRAS

Dedication

I dedicate this book to my family. My dad, who called his daughters "magic." My mom, who raised fearless, compassionate women. My sister, Cathy, who creates safe spaces for her (and other) children—my littlest loves, Kate and Ty. And my dog, Fife, who's probably lying on my feet right now.

I also dedicate this book to the land. I grew up and still live in the province of Alberta. For thousands of years, Blackfoot, Cree, and Métis nations were stewards of the land. European settlers created treaties with these communities, but as a country, we have yet to uphold our end of these agreements. Indigenous communities still do not have adequate access to water, sustenance, or health care that recognizes their traditional ways. As a physician, I'm complicit in upholding the systemic structures that affect Indigenous communities. As a white settler, I don't want to share a superficial land acknowledgment and think that it absolves me of my responsibility. I am committed to truth and reconciliation, as I live on this stolen land and study within a culture that upholds genocide.

Lastly, I dedicate this book to my patients. None of their personal stories are in these pages, but the immense honor I've had of accompanying them on this journey of life has informed my perspectives and the examples that I describe. While I know other doctors have made the choice to relay their patients' experiences without identifying information, my belief is that these stories are unique, need to be handled with delicate care, and are simply not mine to tell. But they live in my heart, which I will open to you here.

Awareness

You've picked up a book with the word *trauma* in the title, so you're aware that some content may trigger unpleasant memories, sensations, and symptoms. If it does, just know these are normal—all of us experience these, some more intensely than others. I hope that you'll find some tools in these pages to help you move through these feelings faster and begin healing. It's all about allowing natural flow.

My perspective is that trauma happens both within individual bodies and our collective consciousness. To me, speaking about trauma also requires us to examine the systems that uphold its causes. As such, I've included content about inequities and social issues, not just teaching about the nervous system. My way of experiencing the world is unique, and so my point of view may not match yours. I don't claim to hold any universal truth, only my own.

I will not be using formal diagnoses or labels like character traits, mental illness, or personality disorders. Personally, I don't believe these are always helpful. Such terms may help find online communities where you can ask questions and share experiences, but I believe that health happens outside of these diagnoses, where we focus on strengths and possibilities.

Let's find out.

Rather than include references in the manuscript or notes at the end, I have compiled notes that I will host online as a living document. I look forward to all of us sharing resources and updating these pages together.

In every chapter, I'll offer practices for you to explore. These practices are experiments where you can choose to try something new—they are invitations, never expectations. Part of the goal of these offerings is to have you notice how you feel before, during, and after each of the activities—to see what works for you. Think of it as something playful and welcoming rather than a prescription. You are the one in charge here.

Introduction

Thank you so much for joining me. You are most welcome.

Imagine we're sitting in the same room together. Would you like it to be a kitchen? Should we share a cup of tea or a warm meal? You'll have to imagine I made it for you, because in real life that would probably be disappointing (my sister is the cook in our family).

Or it could be a living space, with colors you prefer. Maybe a blanket? Would you like it to be weighted? The temperature is just right, and we're sitting a distance apart that feels safe for you.

Safe is the most important part. Safe is key. I'd like you to imagine a space where we are safe together. This is not an office where there's a power dynamic and you might be on edge, feeling diagnosed or dissected. None of that happens here. All you are—is welcome. All you are—is invited. You're the one in control.

Choose the words that feel good for you, that feel right for you. If anything you read here hurts, I am so sorry. My intention is to hold you with incredible awareness and for you to hold yourself with the same. I care about you deeply. I promise you this.

There might be an entire chapter that you'll skip. There might be a paragraph you would like to cross out and rewrite. Please do that. Send it to me. It's important for me to know.

I believe the communities that have been through trauma are the experts. It's been a gift to learn from them for over twenty years. I've also received the gift of learning from the world's greatest experts, where I've studied an alphabet soup of trauma therapies.

I've had the honor of sharing space with people who faced serious challenges as children. People who suffer from the structural violence in society that left them in poverty, often without a home. I've shared time with people who use drugs, who restrict their eating, or use all kinds of distractions to cope with pain. There is no shame here, only love.

Let me share with you first why I chose "The Modern Trauma Toolkit" as the title of this book.

The word *modern* reflects—while I deeply acknowledge there is pain through every generation of humans—that these times are special. Humans have inflicted trauma on one another since early ancestral times, but there's something different about what we're going through right now. Never before has the inequity been so painfully clear, so available to witness through film and media. Through understanding the interconnectedness of all humans, all living beings, and our shared planet. Knowing so many people have a unique existence in the world. Whether they're working in a garment factory in Bangladesh, making fast fashion for pennies. Whether they're an Indigenous elder trying to preserve the rainforest in Brazil. They could be a First Nations person in North America, living on a reservation where rates of infectious disease and suicide are among the highest in the world. Or a transgender teenager living in a small town, where they don't feel welcome in their own home. This modern world hurts in a new way. We all struggle. We all handle our stress differently.

It's also important to address climate change. This is something that impacts us all, but we feel powerless and disconnected from it, because it's such a complex issue. It's already affected our lives: wildfires and smoke that have hit so many neighborhoods, droughts that dry out farms where our food grows, expanding tides that threaten some coastal areas faster than others. My time working at a refugee clinic has shown me that climate refugees have already arrived at my shore, and perhaps yours too. You might be one. I want you to know that I acknowledge the pain of these modern times, when leaders are not making sufficient change to manage these massive challenges. It feels scary to me too. I want you to know I'm meeting you here, in this fear and hopelessness.

I'm using the word *trauma* not because I see people for their vulnerabilities but because I believe in post-traumatic growth. A growth that blossoms from the cracks that feel so painful. I'm going to share more about what I've learned so far in these pages. I hesitate to use words like *resilience*, because terms like these are so often used against individuals and communities that have had to be resilient in order to overcome harmful systems and hierarchies outside of their control. Oppression is something that needs to change at the level of policy and shifting of biases: the patriarchy, which leaves men with more power; the way we see skin color and define it as a race; colonialism and its cousin capitalism, which see us all as consumers and workers rather than the artists or dreamers that we are—all of these things are so deeply problematic. They've caused all of us collective trauma, no matter which side of the privilege we stand on, and need to be considered.

Trauma is a response to events that a human might go through. All living beings encounter difficult times, but we, as humans, experience them deeply because of the way we think. We have an appreciation of our past, how it shapes who we are in the present, and our assumptions about the future.

Because you picked this book up, I would guess that you've experienced some pain in your life. I'm so very sorry about that. Let me use this as an opportunity not to offer you resilience, which could lead you back to your baseline before being hurt, but to grow together, expand, and heal that which has been wounded to transform into something new.

There's a concept in Japan called *kintsugi*. An artisan repairs a piece of broken pottery with gold or silver resin. The idea is that the pottery is more beautiful for having been broken. We can be like that too. This is what I hope for you.

The last word in the title of this book is *toolkit*. It sounds like we could fix your complex parts with a wrench, like I'm commodifying pain, or making trauma therapy something to be completed—and presto, everything's fixed. I don't mean that. What I want to offer you is a personalized menu to explore. It's an invitation to examine some of the healing methods I've learned. I've had the privilege of traveling all over. My sole purpose has been to study as much as I could about healing, to help people who've been through trauma. And I offer this learning to you here. It is incomplete and comes packaged with my personal perceptions. This means that ideally you would notice, really pay attention to your body, and consider which tools feel good and which ones don't. Sometimes trauma takes those instincts away—we'll talk about that too.

The toolkit is yours. You might choose to share it with others. And I would appreciate it if you would also share with me your experiences. I've learned absolutely everything in these pages because of the patients that have chosen a relationship with me and because of the teachers that I have found. I believe that, rather than being an expert in a community, the community is the expert. None of what I offer here is medical advice.

This QR code links to videos with demonstrations of the body-based practices, audio recordings of the mindful practices, color versions of the illustrations, and an opportunity to connect with others—including book club guides. One hope that I have is that we can create a living resource document together—instead of references at the end of this book, I'll keep them updated (with your help) through a document linked here:

(Look at this image through the camera of your smartphone or tablet and tap the image with your finger to get to the page.)

My wish is that you'll become an expert on your own body's response to trauma and that by the end of these pages, we will emerge, forging a path toward post-traumatic growth. This process creates greater possibilities of a hopeful future for us as individuals, who live within a family (chosen or otherwise) and interact in a greater community. I'm deliberately not using the word *empower*, because your power was never mine to give back to you. In fact, you had it all along. I look forward to showing you some places where it might be. We will awaken and enliven together.

Books, health care, and doctors haven't always been safe for all people. I hate that I have to say this, but it's important, and my goal is to create a safe space. I will address racism, transphobia, fatphobia, sexism, ageism, classism, and many other ways that humans have hurt one another. And these human-made concepts create violence. They're not based on any truth, but they uphold existing systems. I will also share some ways in which I have experienced privilege within these systems. Once you finish the book, I hope we can break the harmful systems down together. It may be something you're already working on, but sometimes when your inner pain is so loud, it's hard to bear these larger ones. I hope that we can lessen your inner discomfort, these fire alarms going off in your mind all day, so that we can pay greater attention to some of these larger forces that shape the traumas we face. Our goal is to acknowledge both our ancestors' strengths as well as challenges and to make this world better for the next generations, becoming good ancestors ourselves.

That last phrase, "good ancestors," comes from Indigenous ways of knowing that have been shared with me. I know that because of the power I hold with the title of doctor and with my other social positions, as well as my whiteness, there is a possibility that I could do harm in this book. I'm going to try my best not to.

I want this to be a safe space.

You are welcome here.

AN INVITATION TO EXPLORE

CHAPTER I

Greeting

The Doctor Is In

Let's go through the credentials quickly. I am a family doctor with a master's in medical education. I've studied trauma with the greatest minds in the world, from Gabor Maté to Ruth Lanius to Bessel van der Kolk. And as I write, I'm starting a doctorate at a university in London, England. One research question is how often, throughout my career, have I successfully flipped the traditional power hierarchy: rather than being the expert in the community, how often have I worked with the community as the expert?

It took me a long time of unlearning to know how important this was. So, I'm not writing this book as an expert, although let me assure you I spent years studying all the trauma background and techniques that we're going to explore here. My learning comes from patients who shared their stories, like delicate porcelain that I hold humbly in my hands. My learning comes from communities, like the refugee clinic where I've heard about the most horrifying betrayals and torture that humans can inflict on one another. My learning comes from the people who emerged from the other side, persevering with a faint flicker of hope for a better future.

As much as I see complexity in my experience, it was built on a foundation of collective pain. We uphold so much inequity around the world, where a person like me has hundreds of times more comfort than someone born on the other side of the planet. Or someone born on an Indigenous reservation, living in social and public health conditions much more similar to impoverished countries than the rest of Canada.

I created a residency training in health equity, where student doctors learned how to work with populations of people who face oppression. So, in medicine, yet again, we define humans by their weakness. But I'm hoping that I taught my students to see their patients' strengths and the power of community. These doctors now work with Indigenous people, on and off reserve. They work with Doctors Without Borders (Médecins Sans Frontières, or MSF), helping after natural disasters or war. They work side by side with me at the refugee clinic, teaching me so much about the health of people from Eritrea, Syria, and even Bhutan (a country that attracts attention for measuring gross national happiness, but there are some people experiencing violence from those in power).

I learned about overcoming pain of the past through many patients that have been generous with their stories at the community health centers where I've had the privilege to work. At the addiction clinic, I help people understand that their drug use was a response to the discomfort in their nervous system, responding to traumas that they hold in their body. Once the shame breaks open and allows the light of self-compassion, that's where I learn how much expansion, how much transformation, is possible. It gives me hope for every one of these people, some hope for all humanity.

I learned from you, the reader, many of whom are here because you saw me on TikTok. I showed up there in January 2021, knowing how much trauma and stress were affecting people. But I didn't understand at the time just how incredible the community was there. Mental health creators drop one-minute video clips of brilliance. People share their experiences and wisdom in authentic and fascinating ways. As a therapist, I know that creativity and performance art can heal trauma. The healing on TikTok is awe-inspiring. I see pain and beauty. I hear fears and insights. The longer I follow people, the more I see their growth, their hard work as they shed pain from the past. I see beautiful communities supporting one another through shared experiences and simply caring. Tackling the trolls together, sometimes even sending a TikTok army to right the wrongs in the world. I feel so lucky to have found this community. While I entered the space as a contributor, I found myself once more in the seat of the student. Many of you have been my teacher.

Family Ties

My first teachers were my parents—"You're three-quarters Scottish and a quarter Ukrainian." One of my earliest memories is of my father holding me on his knee, my chubby hands grasped around his fingers. He bounces me with every word, and I remember giggling like it's the funniest thing I'd ever heard. And then he laughs, because he does not know why I think it's funny.

It wasn't until I got older that I realized the significance of what he was saying. I come from somewhere—these places, these people, live in my bones.

I don't have any memories of my dad's parents. It wasn't until I studied trauma when I thought to ask him about his childhood. It turns out he'd never heard the words "I love you" from either of his parents. Speaking to a parent about their own attachment trauma isn't easy; I didn't know where to start.

And now he's gone, so I can't ask.

I was in St. Petersburg, Russia, with my friend Margo, checking out of our hotel. We had just spent two weeks high-altitude camping in Kyrgyzstan, sleeping in yurts on soft, damp mattresses on the floor. But a text from my sister ended the trip.

"Call me. It's dad."

So, I FaceTimed my last good-bye with the person who understood me most in this world. As we sped in a taxi to the airport, I told my dad how much I loved him and that it was okay for him to go if that's what he needed to do.

Six months later, I lost my grandmother. She was hilarious, one of the best storytellers I've known. I started writing because of her stories. But my grandma was so ashamed of her Ukrainian heritage that she never told a single one of her friends outside of her community. She let them believe she was Scottish, like the last name she had taken. Because being a Ukrainian at that time in Alberta (she was born in 1915) meant you faced discrimination; it was presumed Ukrainians were stupid and lazy, though they were hard-working farmers. My curiosity helped my grandmother reshape her story into fondness and pride.

Early into the COVID-19 pandemic in 2020, I got a frantic phone call from my mom, asking me to talk to the ambulance drivers who were in my grandmother's mint-tiled bathroom, where she'd fallen from a major stroke. The EMS gently lifted her birdlike body into her bed and stayed until my mother could come. I arrived with my medical knowledge and an air mattress, spending two days administering medications to keep Grandma comfortable. Murmuring to her, trying to get one last story, one last smile. She wasn't able to eat, and her voice was garbled, so I lost her in pieces before she finally died.

As she passed, I wrapped my legs and arms around her and whispered to her for a minute (or maybe ten) that she was loved.

You are loved. It still echoes within me.

The most challenging part was helping to slide her into the body bag when the funeral home staff came short-handed.

And I was loved. But I wanted you to know that I have suffered significant loss, just in these past two years. Our own traumas are things that we professionals don't talk about. But they shape us. Even the ancestral trauma of my impoverished heritage on both sides. Growing up, I only knew about the Ukrainian traditional foods or the Scottish kilts. There's so much more. There's pain. There's oppression. And I am affected by that, too, without knowing it. I'll speak more to the fact that people suffer compounding trauma—where other factors like race, gender, and class intersect with their experiences. Later, I'll speak to healing traditions and cultural practices. Because there's always wisdom.

I will not spend the rest of this chapter detailing my grief or traumas. But I want you to know something about these parts of me. Not as a physician, but as a human being and my place in this world. Because that matters more than the letters behind my name.

While I had the indescribable sorrow of recently losing two of the people that I loved the most, and within six months of each other, at least I had that love shape me. This abundance of love and care is something I want to offer you as you read this book. My intention is to offer it as a gift, the things I have been privileged to experience, to witness and study. Because I know it helps people.

And while this book is about trauma, it's also about post-traumatic growth. It's also about grit. It's also about gifts.

The Doctor Is Out

As a physician, the only labels I'm allowed to assign people are negative ones. Obesity. Dementia. Illness. Degeneration. With psychiatric conditions, the labels are even more negative, because of the stigma that carries a biased weight with them. It also carries questions. Because the diagnostic manual is constructed from the consensus of a very particular group of people. These diagnoses aren't always endorsed by the community with lived experience. And I now understand that this matters more than a book that tries to put them into little boxes.

Not just them. Not just you. Me too.

When I was studying to get into medical school, I would spend hours in the library. Days bled into one another. After the library was closed at midnight, I found a table outside to keep studying. Highlighter staining my fingers, the whispers of other students were my white noise.

I would drink four cups of coffee, sometimes five or six, to get through those study sessions. Some nights, by the time I got home, I was trembling and my heart was pounding out of my chest. I felt so unwell once, that I phoned the emergency room at the hospital where I was volunteering. As I was sobbing to the nurse that I was definitely having a heart attack, she told me I was actually having a panic attack.

Luckily, I was taking undergraduate psychology at the time.

When I described my symptoms to my professor, the sense of over-whelming doom, he loaned me one of his own books. It described anxiety symptoms and a technique in which I could recognize them and send new signals to my body. I practiced observing my symptoms with an impartial perspective. Reassuring myself that it was an emotion, interpreting my inner sensations, and willing that it would pass. Then, breathing deeply until it did. Eventually, these waves of panic no longer caused the same amount of distress. In these early days as a scientific researcher (we would say $n = 1$, because it was a study on myself of only one participant), I started journaling to investigate the days that the symptoms would be worse. The most extreme anxiety correlated with the days when I drank the most cups of coffee. By the time I stopped drinking anything with caffeine, the panic attacks also slid away. I stopped associating my bed with fear. Which is for-tunate, because I now understand how those kinds of associations could have caused me a lifetime of insomnia, nightmares, and anxiety. This could have left my body stuck in a "trauma response."

I still have anxiety. But I'm not debilitated by psychiatric symptoms any-more. And I understand from my prior experiences, as well as the scientist I've become, just how powerful the mind-body connection is. And honestly, I can't wait to share it with you in this book.

While I have shared some of my vulnerabilities with you, there are more to come. Because I understand my position of privilege in this world. As a physician, people listen when I stand up and advocate. I hold educational, financial, and social power. And I want you to know that I see that too. So, I'm going to come to this writing, as much as I'm capable of, with the lens of curiosity and humility. With the acknowledgment that I've learned so much in the communities where I've had the honor of serving. And I have so much more to learn.

My privilege also comes with responsibility. People like me, with white skin and economic stability, my ancestors were settlers into a country that was built on the genocide of Indigenous people who continue to experience intentional trauma. As an individual, I uphold modern slavery every time I order cheap items on the internet. I contribute to global warming every time I jump on a plane to support the nonprofit work I do.

Understanding is a meager step without action. And so, I use my privilege to give a voice to today's systems-level challenges (like poverty, racism, or discrimination). I have witnessed, at a deep level, how much they impact a person's life and their opportunities. How hard their parents have to work just to put food on the table. They may not get the dad who has time to bounce their baby on his knee like I did. Their dad might work in a meat-packing plant, driving an Uber when he gets home. Their mom might work as a nursing aide in a long-term care center, though she was a nurse in her home country. A traumatized mom might be detached from her children to protect from her own pain. People who experience trauma or detachment in childhood might develop the same coping strategies of their parents, without having access to therapy. I'm just as committed to shifting these structures as I am to the individual harms.

As I share these thoughts with the world, new communities may form around some of these ideas—communities where I can continue to learn. There's so much that we still don't know about the human body and brain's potential. The study of trauma is relatively new within medicine, a field that seeks to define you by the things that are wrong with you. Here—I want to define your experience by what's possible. By what's right with you. By the beauty and potential and innate wisdom that lives within each of us. Because I have learned about this too. And I'm disappointed there's not a diagnostic code for these significant things.

Let's fix the discipline of medicine together, shall we? Imagine if we focused on strengths as well as vulnerabilities. Imagine if we brought all the ancestral and complementary wisdom of the world to bear on every problem. Imagine if we harnessed the power of the mind-body connection to create health instead of treating illness. Imagine if we untangled health care from industries like insurance and pharmaceuticals. Imagine if we all learned from communities living the experiences, from every encounter we would expect to resource one another.

Every person is an expert on their own body. On their own experience. And we physicians, we fail to recognize that so often. Many patients have encountered medical trauma. You might even have trouble trusting me. I understand and I'm sorry that happened to you. Part of why I'm writing this is so that you can see that there is compassion underneath our tender skin. I know in my bones that healing isn't something I learned out of a textbook or during my apprenticeship as a student doctor; it's something I learned as I opened my own heart to truly love my patients. I approach this relationship with humanity rather than expertise—where I come eager to learn, to understand myself as much as others.

LET'S PRACTICE—RIVER OF LIFE

This is an exercise I learned while working at the refugee clinic from a visiting expert on immigrant health. It helps the patients understand that every life has obstacles and beauty.

If you want to do it as an activity, grab a pen or something with which to color. If not, simply use your imagination.

You are welcome to try the River of Life practice.

First, imagine a gently flowing river, the color and size of it. If you're drawing, keep it on a single page.

Next, put the word "birth" and your current age on either end of this river.

Decide when the big events that shaped you took place—don't think about these things in detail, just think of the approximate age when it happened and where that would be on the river.

For challenges (losses, social problems, illnesses), draw a rock or obstruction in or near the river. Decide how big it would be, whether the river flow is blocked.

For joyful life events (knowing that even successes can cause stress), draw a tree or bench alongside the river or some lotus flowers floating on top.

Look back at the river. Can you see that there was difficulty, but also beauty?

RIVER OF LIFE

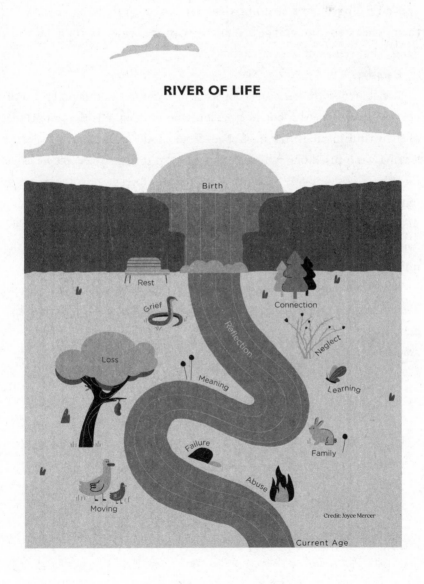

Credit: Joyce Mercer

Let's Spark Something

This book is intended to be one where you take what you need, plant seeds of your own, and grow it into something that's meaningful for your own life context. To share with your friends, neighbors, students, or children. When reading about something that you don't identify or agree with, tell them what's on your mind, or share it with me. None of these ideas are fixed. They're meant to be invitations.

Catalysts.

I've shared with you a sliver of what brought me to this point. I write not just as a physician, but as a person who understands the importance of the vast disparities that have shaped our modern world, that collective trauma has infused our systems and policies so that many people have had their sense of safety taken from them by greater forces. So, while there's so much that can be done within your body to heal from trauma, the systems that uphold these structural inequities and violent global injustices remain. And so, I hope that we also, as a society, continue to work to dismantle this imbalance.

But first, I want to invite you to continue to turn the pages while we take a strength-based approach to trauma. Because I see not just the wounds that people have suffered, I see the beauty of the light that shines through those cracks.

CHAPTER 2

Trauma

Humans have been through awful times—wars, famine, weather catastrophes, and pandemics. Our day-to-day lives are often stressful and challenging. It's safe to say that many of us have been through trauma. Some people differentiate, calling an experience "big T" or "little T" traumas, which makes many people feel invalidated.

But what is trauma?

It doesn't matter what specific events you've gone through. It only matters how your body handles it, in terms of whether something has been traumatic.

Trauma is not the thing that happened. It's the body's response to that experience. Gabor Maté speaks beautifully to this.

Sometimes the trauma is something that's missing, like neglect or compassion.

Brain Evolution

Every human body is also a mammal, a warm-blooded animal. So, just like dogs and horses and even elephants, we handle stress biologically. And, just like these animals, our body is designed to process stress. Think of how these beautiful creatures always seem to sense the emotions of other animals around them. Has a dog ever licked your tears? Mine sure has. Have you ever watched a dog or a horse shake their whole body when they're stressed? (It turns out that humans can do this too.) Elephants grieve when one is lost.

How our body handles trauma is to remind us about it, to protect us from something similar happening again in the future. The brain thinks about the event and the context (like time of day, weather, or location). And it constantly scans the environment, looking for things that are related. The amygdala, or "fire alarm center" of the brain, sends out a warning signal whenever it detects something that reminds it of this dangerous memory. These are experienced as uncomfortable flashbacks, nightmares, and triggers.

Triggers can be anything that reminds the brain of the event—a sound or a smell, running into a person or seeing them on social media. Even a word or a feeling will do it. Then, the warning signal creates behaviors, so fast it's like a reflex. Our brain wires these patterns in and preferentially chooses that path. When it happens often enough, this gets interpreted as personality traits.

So, why are we designed this way?

To prevent something bad from happening, we learn from the times that it's happened in the past. Our brain has a special storage area that helps us learn about dangerous scenarios and sends reflex signals out to the rest of our body to prepare us or to help us avoid the problem. It's important to understand that the mechanism that reacts to trauma is not our enemy. It's not meant to be harmful or distressing, though it's sometimes experienced that way. These responses are there to protect us.

Clinical Definitions

The American Psychological Association defines *trauma* as "an emotional response to a terrible event." While I appreciate they say it's the response and not the event that causes trauma, I'm not convinced that it's purely emotional.

How would that explain why a body tenses up, the heart pounds, and the skin breaks into a sweat—when reminded of the experience?

The response, in my view, is one that takes place in the entire nervous system. The connection between the brain and the body.

The book that psychiatrists follow is called *The Diagnostic and Statistical Manual of Mental Disorders*, fifth edition, commonly known as the DSM-5. This medical text describes trauma narrowly—only "death, serious injury, and sexual violence" qualify in the DSM-5 as traumatic events. The psychiatrists who wrote the most recent version of this book decided these scenarios could happen to ourselves, to those we love, as something we've witnessed, or as part of our job—to cause trauma. According to the psychiatric textbooks, even if you have all the classic symptoms of post-traumatic stress disorder (PTSD), it would only count if you were exposed to these exact scenarios. This leaves out many people I've met who have traumatic responses because of a chronic illness, severe bullying, or abusive parents. It fails to mention discrimination, birth trauma, and ancestral trauma—many things we now know affect people in subconscious ways. The psychiatry textbook defines the trauma as the event, not the way the body responds to it.

The DSM-5 does, however, include a helpful definition of how trauma shows up in the body. I will not go through the whole checklist, because it's very clinical and academic, but it's worth knowing about the categories:

1. Intrusive Symptoms

This sounds exactly like the word—thoughts and emotions, or even physical symptoms, intrude in a person's life. They jump in unexpectedly. The thoughts appear as nightmares, flashbacks, and painful memories. They show up uninvited. And they terrorize.

Why the Brain Thinks This Helps

If you think about it, intrusive symptoms serve a purpose after trauma. They're a constant reminder of the things to avoid. It's like having a sign on the entrance to a door into something awful—Do Not Enter. The brighter and more obvious the sign, the more likely you'll notice it.

Here's an Example

Alex tosses and turns in bed more than he sleeps. His sister died in a house fire, and he can't stop thinking about it. He blames himself because she was in the next room. He's never told his parents, but he showed his sister how to use a lighter, and she must have found the one Alex used for smoking. Every time he smells smoke, images of the fire play like a movie, and he hears his sister's screams.

2. Avoidance Symptoms

This looks like a person who doesn't leave their house very often. Or doesn't go to any places that remind them of their past. They avoid people who might be triggering. Ultimately, they spend a lot of energy to avoid being exposed to something that might be painful.

Why the Brain Thinks This Helps

This makes sense, too, in terms of protection. If you can stay away from a situation that could cause pain, then you can prevent it from happening. Protection is enhanced when you don't run into any external triggers at all.

Here's an Example

Kaile hasn't left her room in three days but sneaks out at night to graze on snacks in the kitchen. It's important she doesn't see anyone who was at the party where she blacked out. She's pretty sure someone spiked her drink, but doesn't want to think about who or why. Kaile doesn't feel like dealing with anyone in her family; they keep asking her what's wrong, but she doesn't want to talk about it. She doesn't answer her friends' text messages except with one or two words and hasn't gone out with them in weeks, though it's summer break. She spends her time on Instagram, looking at baking videos and knitting tips. She doesn't do either of those things.

3. Depressive Symptoms

The DSM-5 describes this as a feeling of low mood and having negative thoughts. It can also show up as a lack of motivation, being tired and feeling blah, being moody or irritable. It's commonly experienced as a brain fog, having trouble concentrating (even reading), or not being able to remember things. Extreme versions show up as being numb and not feeling much at all.

WHY THE BRAIN THINKS THIS HELPS

Depressive symptoms are the brain's way of "checking out" when it feels overwhelmed. When it's been putting in too much energy, this helps it slow down. It seems counterintuitive, because depression is stressful and uncomfortable, but the body can't stay in the "alert mode" for very long. It gets tired and needs a rest.

HERE'S AN EXAMPLE

Jayde tried to get a part-time job for two months, turning in applications at all the retail and fast-food places that he could bike to. Two of the managers told him he'd have to cut his braids to work there, which he'd never do. One told him he wouldn't fit in. He knew what they meant. There wasn't a single Black employee at that store. Rent is due, but he can't leave the apartment to keep trying. He rewatches movies and plays video games, trying not to think about it. He doesn't feel like making music anymore, or even eating, because it just doesn't matter. His life is turning out just like his older brothers', though he swore it would never happen to him. He feels so hopeless that he wakes up crying.

4. Reactive Symptoms

The technical word for this is *hypervigilant*, which means that a person is always on the alert for threats. They scan the outside world for danger. They notice every little sound or stranger. They might have trouble being in crowds. If someone touches their shoulder, they might jump because they startle easily. They might position themselves in a room so they can see the door, watching who comes in or out.

WHY THE BRAIN THINKS THIS HELPS

This active "alert mode" is like a fire alarm. It's a great warning system to let you know something dangerous is nearby. But this fire alarm is set to be too sensitive, so it goes off with a whiff of smoke. And it's really loud, so it demands a lot of attention.

HERE'S AN EXAMPLE

Ryan can't study in the library because every noise makes her startle. She tries to read with headphones on, but then she can't hear if someone is approaching and ends up always looking behind her. One time, a car backfired, and she actually screamed. That was embarrassing. When she studies in her house, she plays music in the background to keep her mind from wandering. Every time her stomach growls, she tells herself she has colon cancer, just like her dad did. She is so worried that her stepmom will find out where she lives, so she dyed her hair blond and takes a route to her university that is ten minutes out of the way. When she sees a red-haired woman, she turns in the other direction and walks as fast as she can. She's never going back to that house.

5. Risk-Taking

One symptom that was controversial to include in the latest version of the DSM-5 was that of reckless behavior: someone takes a lot of risks and doesn't seem to care about the chances they take. This was a small subgroup of people after trauma, but enough of the psychiatrists felt that it was important to mention.

WHY THE BRAIN THINKS THIS HELPS

If you think about it, dangerous activities would distract you from inner emotional pain. When you have to concentrate hard to survive, when your body is experiencing extreme danger—this takes a lot of energy and attention away from other types of pain.

Another reason this might show up is *congruence*. When the outside world matches your insides (your nervous system is ramped up, as it should be when you're in danger), then the world might make more sense. Think: "Of course my heart is pounding and I'm scared. I'm jumping out of a plane!"

HERE'S AN EXAMPLE

Gil started racing dirt bikes when his mom went to jail. He loved the speed of it; the wind whipping his hair and his teeth cold from smiling. He especially liked when he could bump the other riders off the course; that felt so satisfying. After a while, he converted to BMX bikes and got a reputation for being fearless. He'd jump higher and longer than anyone else on the track, sometimes not even on a bet. One time, he broke his collarbone and some ribs when he landed on the bike. He can't wait until he's eighteen and can start racing cars. He's already taken his dad's car out at night and drag-raced it downtown. The last time, he saw a cop car and turned home in a panic. Luckily, his dad and the new girlfriend don't notice as long as he puts the keys back in the exact same place. The punishment would be intense, but that risk is piled on top of all the others.

LET'S PRACTICE—THE RADIO

Your brain gets constant signals from what's going on inside and around your body. After trauma, it tends to pay more attention to these signals, checking for threats.

Think of this as a bunch of radio and streaming stations.

Your brain will tune into a station if it seems important, giving it news that it needs.

It may turn the volume dial way up, to hear it better.

The next time your brain is ruminating (overthinking) about something specific, how can you:

- Turn down the volume
- Change stations
- Not let the chatter bother you

Having all the radio stations playing at once is overwhelming.

But you can learn to play them only as loud as you can handle.

Imagine turning a huge volume dial down in your mind. You may choose to mimic the idea, twisting your ear or nose. Imagine a radio that's blaring and how much of a relief it is to have it become quieter.

Could you imagine silence?

Trauma Criteria

There's no shared definition about what makes something traumatic. As we just learned, it's not the event, but the response, that matters.

Trauma is not something that happens outside the body. It's the body's response to the things that happen, trying to keep you safe. The body has intelligence, just like your brain. Even when the responses to perceived threats don't always seem smart or helpful, your body is doing its best to interpret the information it's receiving and try to protect you.

What kinds of situations create a traumatic response in the mind?

1. Trauma Changes Our World

Trauma makes a person feel that the world is different. That it's not as predictable as they'd hoped. They feel it's possible to be threatened, physically or emotionally. That someone they love or care for could be at risk or could harm them.

The most common thing I've heard, working with people who've been through something traumatic, is that they no longer feel that the world is a safe place.

They don't trust in things to "be okay." They don't trust that "the universe has their back."

This belief changes a lot of pathways in the brain. When you don't believe the world is safe, you plan your day differently. You're on edge, looking for danger. When you don't believe the world is safe, you often have difficulty trusting new people. Or even the ones you know.

2. Trauma Is Unexpected

Think about a natural disaster—an earthquake, major fire, or a hurricane—that will cause a traumatic reaction for many people caught in it. It's scary in the moments when it happens. But once you've survived, your body will always be on guard for something else to happen again. You'll pay more attention to weather reports and cloud formations.

After I survived the series of massive earthquakes in Nepal in 2015, certain physical cues can trigger my trauma response. If I'm in a building with a garage and the door opens, so the building shakes, that's a reminder. The sound of a plate breaking, just like it did in my apartment in Nepal that afternoon, is an extra-loud shatter for me. Traumatic reactions turn up the volume dial compared to another person experiencing the same situation.

Something else that would make the trauma unexpected is if the person who causes it is in a position of trust. If it's a stranger, that could be a police officer, but it can also be a teacher or an employer.

Being Black or Indigenous can feel dangerous around people in authority positions. You never know who might be racist and cause you serious harm. While I suggest the situation is unexpected, it's more that it doesn't have to be dangerous to be traumatic—the trauma responses can show up in anticipation. But especially for certain oppressed communities, it often is dangerous too.

In many cases, the most damaging person that causes trauma is a parent, which is unexpected and scary for a child. This sets the body up for something we call *developmental* or *attachment* trauma. When someone was not safe that really should have been, it changes the foundational beliefs held in the body. You feel that the world is not safe. The people who should have protected you didn't. That kind of hurt runs deep, often showing up subconsciously in the adult body or relationships.

3. Trauma Is Faced Alone

There are two ways to look at this aspect of trauma.

The positive way is to remember that, if we do not face the stress alone, that is protective. If we have a safe person to go to—a sibling, a friend, a teacher, a neighbor—that often means that the problem we face doesn't lay down significant trauma pathways in the brain afterward.

Things don't always work out that way.

Sometimes, horrible events happen when we're alone.

Sometimes, a scary person involved tells us we can't share the secret.

Sometimes, we don't want to share because we can't find the words or we feel ashamed.

When something happens and we feel isolated when we deal with it, that's more likely to cause a future trauma response.

Complex Trauma

Anyone who's had more than one traumatic response happen in different circumstances would be diagnosed with complex trauma.

There are many people who work in the trauma field that would suggest anything that happens to you as a child would fall into this category. This developmental or attachment trauma involves a young child and their inter-actions with parents or caregivers. Or, let's be clear about this, the people who are supposed to give care. They often can't or don't.

I know it's hard to imagine this about people who cause harm, but it's truly the case that most of them had a great deal of trauma when they were kids too. Hurt people might hurt others, unless they process the trauma they've been through and gain distance from the reflex responses. It's hard to be a parent when you never knew what safe parenting looked like from your own childhood.

Everyone's doing the best they can. I believe that. But this doesn't stop them from being accountable to the pain they might inflict.

It's incredible how often I'm working with someone and discussing what their body's trauma response looks like. Then, they have a conversation with a parent that had always been aloof or threatening, only to find out their parent's trauma story. It doesn't make the behavior okay, but it helps us show more compassion toward why it happened—which helps the feeling of shame. Knowing why it happened helps you know that you never, ever, even a little bit, deserved it.

Complex trauma is not a universally defined medical term. It didn't get accepted into the DSM-5. We didn't learn about it in medical school. It's not a diagnosis that can go on your chart (yet).

But that doesn't mean it's not a genuine state.

How to Be Trauma-Informed

Given how many people have experienced trauma, and you don't know what their triggers might be, how do you approach people with care so as not to re-create their trauma response? That's what we call being *trauma-informed*. A new way of speaking about it, so as not to focus on the negative, is *healing-centered engagement*. I like this because it shows what you want rather than what you don't want.

Here are some ideas:

I. Watch the Tone of Voice

Lots of research shows that the way you speak to someone is almost as important as what you say. *Vocal prosody* describes a melodic voice that moves from low to high pitch smoothly. The way the ear hears this sound is relaxing and can change the nervous system state.

Likewise, raising the voice or speaking in a flat monotone can be interpreted as unsafe. That's not the fault of the person speaking. It's just the way the nervous system works. There's likely a connection to the person who births, where having more estrogen hormone often means the voice has more of this quality. It's why toddlers or dogs can be more leery of male-identifying people.

2. Show Vulnerability

When the situation feels safe for you, being authentic about your own struggles can be a powerful way to help a person feel safe dealing with theirs. Reflecting on the interaction creates an open door for them to relax.

"I know you didn't mean to, I always know you're doing the best you can, but when you say that I'm stomping around, it makes me feel like I'm bothering you. Is there something else going on? Sometimes when I hear loud noises, it makes me nervous."

You don't necessarily want them to open up and talk about their trauma. That can be hard to hear about—your own brain might feel overwhelmed (we call this *vicarious trauma*), or you might not feel equipped to help. Especially if a person doesn't have the tools and resources to be aware of their traumatic response and manage it—at the end of the conversation, they can feel worse.

Allowing yourself to show a range of emotions—being real about when you're sad, when you're angry, when you're frustrated, when something has triggered you—can be healing for a person who feels these emotions to the extreme.

3. Watch for Cues

When you think someone's acting strangely, ask yourself if it's a trauma response.

The minute the question pops into your head, "What's wrong with that person? They're—rude, weird, irritating, inconsistent—[or insert another description]." Trauma can show up in all of those ways.

Imagine a body is stuck in alert mode. That person will seem jumpy, angry at minor things, or eager to misinterpret something said. This is because every signal their brain gets is assumed to be dangerous.

A tap on the shoulder? Likely bad news, so the body becomes quickly afraid. The person twists or jumps away. That can be hurtful if it's a close friend or a love interest.

Being told a rule, like "wear a mask at the store" as a public health order to prevent spread of a virus? Instant catastrophe, a sense that it will stop them from being able to breathe.

A comment that could be seen as accusing will be carried to the extreme. "You didn't take out the garbage" becomes "You're a bad person" to the brain that's heard this story before.

Shame is a powerful storyteller.

Now, imagine a body stuck in a numb response. This person will seem like they don't care, like they can't look after themselves, like they can't be reliable. Their body isn't letting them connect anymore; it's too afraid.

> How might you look at the interactions you have in a day differently with this lens?

I'm not encouraging you to accept these behaviors. Set boundaries around the behaviors with people you know so it's clear that you won't accept some of these actions. Just understand where they're potentially coming from. Have the conversation from a place of compassion and love. Always know that it's not your fault.

But it's likely not theirs either.

Post-Traumatic Growth

Resilience is like a rubber band. After you stretch it, wrap it around things, it returns to the same shape.

Likewise, when you've been through trauma, and the system gets through it, whether it's a human body or an animal body or a city—it can return to the same approximate shape.

But if you stretch a rubber band too much, it gets kind of saggy. It might look warped or frayed on one side. It might look frail enough that you wouldn't want to try to stretch it too much again, because it might break.

All the stretching is like compounded trauma. This is why I don't like using the metaphor of resilience, because your only options are to be misshapen or to snap.

Post-traumatic growth is like a Slinky. If you don't know what a Slinky is, it's a coil of wire that can bend in any direction. You can stretch it out from one end of the room to the other. And if you're positioning it just right, on the edge of a step, it can slink right down the stairs.

Post-traumatic growth is like the Slinky because it can return to the shape from before trauma but also take on all kinds of new shapes. That's when you learn all that you're capable of. It's when you stretch, growing far more than your initial starting point would have deemed possible.

Let's use a different metaphor, with a visual. Think of a person as floating through life, then a traumatic event hits them like a wave. They end up underwater, uncomfortable and afraid. Once they build, or are thrown, a

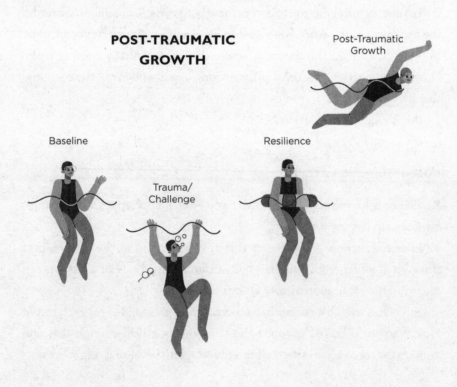

POST-TRAUMATIC GROWTH

Post-Traumatic Growth

Baseline

Resilience

Trauma/ Challenge

flotation device, they spend more time at the surface, which is status quo. That's resilience. When you can swim—that's post-traumatic growth.

The aim of this book is to help you find skills, tools, and concepts to move toward post-traumatic growth. To get you feeling like you've "leveled up." That the trauma has catalyzed a wave of expansion and awareness that's only possible because you've gone through the challenge.

It's my sincere belief that this is the way humans evolve.

CHAPTER 3

Polyvagal Theory

This is probably one of the most important chapters in the book. While I recommend skipping some sections that don't interest you, don't resonate, or don't apply—this is meant to be a "choose your own healing adventure"—I wouldn't skip this one.

The polyvagal theory was created by a scientist, Dr. Stephen Porges, back in the 1980s. He was doing scientific research in a lab and discovered properties about an important nerve, one that Resmaa Menakem (a body-based therapist and "cultural trauma navigator") calls the *soul nerve*.

The vagus nerve—not Vegas like the city—is something I learned about in medical school. I learned it was cranial nerve number ten (*cranial* means "head," so a nerve that goes from the brain to head structures). When we learned how to test if it's working properly, they taught us to make a person gag with a tongue depressor. We will watch your soft palate—the roof of your mouth—to make sure that when you say "ah," it lifts both sides at the same time.

But this nerve does so much more. It's a critical factor in mental health.

Sadly, that's not something I learned in medical school.

The polyvagal theory takes the shame away from mental health issues. It reassures you that the symptoms you notice and the distress that you feel are a part of normal human physiology. It's your body trying to protect you. Often, it's just overprotective.

While there are some controversies related to the theory, I find it an excellent explanation of how trauma shows up and connects the mind with the body. The people who prefer to overlook the theory might be unaware of how useful it is in clinical practice.

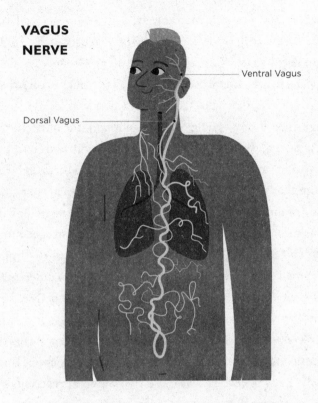

VAGUS NERVE

Ventral Vagus

Dorsal Vagus

Let me show you how it works.

Your vagus nerve goes up into your face, like I was describing. It's in charge of your facial expressions and tone of voice. This is important, because when we are interacting with others, these are the cues we use to decide if they're safe. If they're genuine or caring. We look at their mouth to see if their smile is real—how many teeth they're showing. We look at their eyes for narrowing or a raised eyebrow.

One of the most important factors for safety in the polyvagal theory is tone of voice. A motherly singsong voice is a soothing way to talk to most people, especially those who've been through trauma. So, when I'm in session, and when I'm on TikTok or out in the world, I'm careful about how my voice sounds.

These characteristics influenced by the vagus nerve—facial expression and tone of voice—help us decide if a person is trustworthy. And the rest of our brain decides if we can relax around them. Dr. Porges calls this our *ventral vagus* response—the word *ventral* means "front." So, it's the front of our body—our face—that helps us decide if a person is safe.

The vagus nerve keeps going to the diaphragm, the huge muscle under your heart and lungs that helps you breathe. This is why heart rate (how fast it beats) is a crucial way to tell the state of your nervous system and why breath can influence that state. We'll go into these possibilities in later chapters.

This part of the vagus nerve sends signals to the heart, telling it to slow down (or, as recent research suggests, preventing it from speeding up). Dr. Porges calls this the *vagal brake*. Your heart has a natural rhythm; it's controlled by a small collection of cells that set the pace that's different for every person. It's even different minute to minute. When the body is stressed, it changes the way the vagus nerve sends its signals.

This directs two different trauma responses. Dr. Porges calls them different evolutionary adaptations, but I'm not as certain about this part of the theory. What I believe is that these two different reactions from our brain and vagus nerve create the two different trauma responses that we all default to when stress hits.

The first is familiar to many of us.

High Activation—Sympathetic Nervous System

The fight-or-flight response means that we want to fight off or run away from a problem. You can imagine how this was something adaptive when mammals were roaming. If a predator is chasing you, these are your best chances of escape.

But, in modern times, sometimes the thing that is causing us stress can't be eliminated in this way. It could be your boss or your teacher. It could be a stack of bills you can't pay. It could be your screaming baby reminding you of the siblings you had to raise because your mom wasn't around. It could be living in a dangerous neighborhood. Or it could be experiencing racism as the only Asian kid in your school.

This response is the one that goes through our activating nervous system—called the *sympathetic nervous system*. I like to think of it as giving us sympathy and helping us get out of trouble. In fact, this part of our body is active anytime we have to move. When we clap our hands, walk, type, or sing—the sympathetic nervous system helps us move our muscles. It recruits energy, blood flow with oxygen, to the muscles that need to do the task.

This nervous system activates the heart, to pump nourishing blood around the entire body. It activates part of the brain, whatever is needed most. The sympathetic nervous system keeps your eyes focused on your surroundings (your pupils get wider to let in more light). It also sends energy to the muscles so they can be ready to move.

In prioritizing these parts of the body, other areas like the gut and immune system don't get as much attention. It's hard to sleep when our body is in this activated state; our mind also becomes busy and prone to overthinking. You might experience racing thoughts—generally the regrets of the past and the worries about the future. They play like a radio station that won't turn off in your brain. The brain is scrambling to make sense of what's happening to you. It's not your enemy; it's just trying to create a story so it can work to protect you, based on the information from that story.

What if we thought of it as "protection" instead of "rumination"?

> In Dan Siegel's hand model of the brain, our limbic system (emotion center) is our thumb. If you tuck it into a fist, when the emotions get "too big," it will flip your fingers up. This represents losing our thinking brain. He calls this "flipping our lid."

The sympathetic nervous system gets a terrible reputation. It's essential for our life; we wouldn't be able to move without it. Any movement at all involves this part of our nervous system. We need to move our muscles and keep our heart beating. So, it's not like we want to turn the sympathetic system off.

We just don't want it to be activated to such an extent that it doesn't allow for the flexibility of using other parts of our body. And we don't want it to get stuck in the "full-on" position, where the amount of readiness to move leaves our muscles tense, our mind racing, and our heart pounding. That's exhausting.

HERE'S AN EXAMPLE

Harjit can't stop thinking about her cousin, who came back from a summer trip to India married to a man she'd never met, from the village her mom grew up in. Now, Harjit's parents have booked a family trip to India over her next vacation. She's afraid they might make her marry some old guy. Harjit wakes up in a sweat most nights, whether or not she remembers the nightmare. She feels her heart pounding and a pulse in her temple when she's trying to concentrate at work. Sometimes, the sensation is so intense that she goes to the washroom and splashes water on her face. She can't stop thinking about the upcoming trip, how she has to keep her own passport and find the embassy in case something bad happens. She's irritable with her parents but too scared to confront them. She keeps remembering a time when she was younger, when her mom said to her, "You just think a love match is best. But these boys here, they wouldn't be suitable." Since then, she's had to hide if she's dated anybody. Her boyfriend doesn't know what she's going through; she thinks breaking up with him might save everyone some stress. Every time he comes near her lately, Harjit tenses her shoulders until she gets a headache. She's jumpy with her younger brother; if he knocks on her bedroom door, she startles and screams at him.

The Shift—Connection

If I were to work with Harjit, we'd start by helping her stay safe during sessions by first acknowledging that I'm listening and that I care. It's hard to get yourself out of fight-or-flight when you aren't in a calm body. Then, we'd find out about her physical sensations and use body-based techniques (breath, energy, or touch) to help her come out of such strong activation. She would become the expert at knowing when she's in "fight-or-flight," helping herself shift so it's not as intense. Something as simple as swallowing water or going to the washroom can shift the balance between nervous system states, since it's the calmer nervous system in charge of the digestive tract. Once her body feels more comfortable, we can use brain-based tools (talking about problems and solutions), because her mind would come "back online." We can examine the truth behind her fears. Would her parents really do that? And, if so, what can be done to keep her safe?

The key to healing the high-activation response is connection. With others, with pets, with nature. With ourselves. The more we are connected and present, the more this grounding settles the restless energy.

Low Activation—Dorsal Vagal

When the sympathetic nervous system gets too tired, this is when the low-activation *parasympathetic nervous system* response kicks in. Just as you'd imagine, when any part of our body gets exhausted, it shuts down.

This "shut-down" response, known as *dorsal vagal*, is another way that trauma shows up.

This is the less understood trauma response. It looks like paralysis, feeling stuck and not able to get things done. Not caring about ordinary life. Having no energy to work or study. No energy to spend time with friends and family.

The body often feels sluggish. Muscles feel limp and frail. Everything moves slowly, like it's crawling through mud. The brain is foggy; memory and concentration suffer. Many illnesses include this constellation of symptoms. So, once a doctor like me has evaluated that it's not a medical disease, I would wonder about stress. It could be a sign that the sympathetic nervous system has burned out.

When we discussed the vagus nerve, I mentioned it goes down toward the diaphragm. Here, most of its job is to report to your brain about your body—what sensations you're having, what position you're in, what your internal organs are doing.

If the vagus nerve is not working properly, those signals can be too strong (chronic pain, irritable bowel, and pelvic issues can result). It can also malfunction by slowing the body down too much.

Here's an Example

Ella saw somebody who looked familiar on the subway. Just the way he sat reminded her of her cousin who had hurt her when she was younger. The more she stared at him, the more convinced she became. She felt so heavy in her seat, like she was frozen, that she missed her stop. After the stranger got off the train, Ella still felt outside of her body, almost like she was looking down on it. She rode all the way to the end of the line, and even then it took her some time to figure out how to get home. She's missed three days of work because she just can't get out of bed. Sometimes, she cries—sometimes she just stares at her phone.

The Shift—Movement

If I were to work with Ella, we would first notice the slow feelings in her body. Moving toward small amounts of activation, ones that feel safe for her, would be the first place to start. I like to begin with the imagination. We might use a metaphor, thinking of her cat asleep in a sunbeam. The stillness here isn't painful or threatening, it just is. Then, we would imagine her cat stretching until it has the energy to jump up on the windowsill. Next, we explore what would feel safe and possible for Ella. Getting more active on her phone, texting friends or creating some content for social media. Petting her cat and noticing how it purrs on her chest. Spending a bit more time making food, and then experiencing each bite through the taste and texture.

Just getting out of the trauma experience for a few moments is helpful. And then, when she feels ready, go for a walk outside and notice all the surrounding things. The trees, the dogs on leashes, the colors of each car. The clouds in the sky and how they are rolling, flowing across—exactly how every emotion passes. These mindful steps, moving toward more activation, will help her shift away from this trauma state. Ella might start with moving her big toe. A small activity can be enough to get unstuck.

LET'S PRACTICE—THE LADDER

This is a modification of an exercise created by Deb Dana, the social worker who has brought many of Dr. Porges's ideas into clinical practice.

Imagine that you're climbing a ladder. It could also be the side of a building or a vine. At the bottom of the ladder, your feet are stuck in the mud, and it takes some energy to free them (the bottom is the low-activation state).

To get moving up the ladder, you need to spend some energy (in the high-activation state), but if you climb too high or too fast, you can get tired and slide back down. If this happens, you get more stuck in the mud because you're too exhausted to get moving again.

Once you get to the top, you can rest. You have views of what's around and you can breathe comfortably.

Draw out the ladder or other tall structure—a tree, even a beanstalk. There is an illustration of the ladder on page 178.

Where are you on this—right now? Stuck in the mud? Climbing? How tired does this make you? Or are you resting at the top?

This is the *dorsal vagal* to *sympathetic* to *ventral vagal* progression.

The more you notice your state, the more you can learn tools to shift it.

The Window

Once a person spends more time in the ventral vagal state, they have reached something called the Window of Tolerance, a concept described by a psychiatrist named Dr. Dan Siegel. If you're stuck in the overactive or underactive states of the body, this is stealing a lot of your energy. So, there isn't much energy left for memory and concentration. While you don't need your full thinking brain to process trauma, you need some of it.

Within the Window of Tolerance, you feel you can handle what's going on in front of you. The goal of all therapy with a person who has trauma reflexes is to learn how to spend more and more time in this Window.

How we work through trauma to get to this Window often takes specific steps. I'm going to list them sequentially because the first ones are foundational to the next ones happening. But, like this book, it doesn't have to be happening exactly in this order. Everyone's experience is different and valid.

1. Comfort

In the courses where I studied trauma, it relates to *attunement*. I like this word because being in tune is a little bit like hearing a pleasant instrument. When something is out of tune, it can be jarring. So, this comfort comes from within your own body, being able to experience a state of calm. More important, when you're working with a comforting therapist, it means that you trust them enough to relax in their presence sometimes. If you're not quite in the Window, at least you're on the edge.

Much of this "comfort" step comes from noticing which of the polyvagal states your body is in and shifting it just enough so that you can get closer to calm. I like to help people examine their situation from first-, then second-, then third-person perspectives. With your memories, it would mean being able to look back from your own point of view, as the main character, then as the person you're interacting with, and finally as a person who's watching the overall scene. The more distance, the less pain is reexperienced.

2. Skills Building

Part of what helps all people spend more time in this Window of Tolerance is learning the best pathways for their body. This means paying attention to when you're feeling hyperactivated or not activated enough. I've dedicated the entire second half of this book to the tools I've learned that I'm hoping will help you. But you are the expert on what's working, which is why you are in charge of choosing to explore the ones that bring you closer to this Window.

I call this stage Shifting. Because you're learning how to shift between the nervous system states on your own. This phase of the work takes time, a lifetime really. I don't think of working with trauma as a destination, but as a journey. One that I am on myself, and one that I am on alongside you now.

3. Trauma Processing

Personally, I think you can use trauma-processing skills to manage your day-to-day stress. But for the big traumas, the ones that happened in childhood or the ones that changed your life forever, I recommend the safety of a professional therapist. Safety is so important to me, and though I understand that there might be barriers to access, like time or money, this is the safest thing I can suggest.

Processing trauma means that you reexperience pieces of it, but it doesn't mean you have to talk about it. In the best trauma therapy I know, Accelerated Resolution Therapy (ART), you move your eyes from side to side while watching a movie in your mind about the worst times you've experienced. By the end of the session, you've established new memory associations and emotions to overlay the movie, so triggers and flashbacks melt away. You can remember traumatic events without reexperiencing the pain of those moments. It's the most magical thing I've ever seen. I wish this kind of magic for you, but it's not something that's possible to do on your own. Some elements that it uses, specifically creativity and metaphor, which are the language of the subconscious mind, are aspects I will describe and explore later.

4. Post-Traumatic Growth

This is when you can look back on all the skills that you've learned, new patterns you've formed, and how you've emerged from these traumas. I think these skills, concerning staying in the Window of Tolerance and processing traumatic events, are foundational to human existence and evolution. Some patients that I work with, when they explore post-traumatic growth, end up leaving their profession and serving others in the same way. These exceptional students become my teachers, and often teach others. It's another thing I wish for you, not just to be helped by what you are reading here, but to share your experience.

Everyone's body is different, everyone's context is different, and so I write from my perspective. The more that you can distance yourself from the pain of the past, the more fully you will experience your present.

I think of these steps as gathering resources. Which is why I've mentioned the ones that I think have the best chance of helping you. Although there are some parts of trauma processing that will not come across on the page, I'm excited to share some of these theories and practices with you. Examples of the shifting skills and ways of changing your relationship with the past will enhance your ability to stay calmer in the present.

While I don't share specific opinions about psychiatric medications within this book, they have helped people that I've worked with stay in a calm enough body to learn these skills. The medications aren't the cure in trauma processing, but they can help you explore the ways of being in the world that will feel safe in the future. If a medication is useful to stay in your Window of Tolerance, so that your brain has enough clarity to learn the ways to keep calm more often, then that may be the best path for you.

The entire goal of this work is to develop *mental flexibility*. Once you've experienced trauma, the brain goes down the path toward the traumatic responses of the fight, flight, or freeze symptoms. Once you develop mental flexibility, more pathways are available to you.

Think of it like a place in the jungle where animals and people have been stomping down one path to a cliff. The more new pathways that you can open, the more states of being that you can explore: waterfalls, immense trees, rivers. A brain might choose the familiar path, even if it's toward a trigger event (a dark cave), or a flashback (a bear) when the trauma gets reexperienced with all of its pain. Post-traumatic growth is when the path forward leads to somewhere safe and in the direction that you prefer to explore. A path to a turquoise mountain lake reflecting the majesty behind it, the sun glittering on the surface. A path to a bird's nest. You choose your destination, somewhere beautiful and meaningful.

I believe the purpose of human existence is to find connection and meaning. Connection doesn't necessarily mean a love relationship; it can be connection to the path of our own life and connection to our inner workings. Many people don't spend a lot of time exploring that. Once you feel connected to yourself in that way, you offer yourself friendship and support. In one therapy technique, Internal Family Systems (IFS), your inner parts actually look after one another. The parts who stay in the Window of Tolerance can help the ones who are still stuck in suffering—often the child parts who got stuck in a stress response after something bad happened.

This is some of the resolution that I believe is possible and helps us connect better to others.

Meaning doesn't always come from just the job that you have or art that you make. Learning the skills of keeping your emotions in the Window of Tolerance, and processing stressful situations, can provide immense meaning. I think it's one of the most important paths for humans to explore. I wish they taught stress management in schools!

While I've always appreciated the gifts of the job that I have, it wasn't until I started doing this kind of work with people that my cup of meaning absolutely overflowed. And I know once you connect to it yourself, maybe share it with others, it will become part of what brings you a sense of purpose.

The work of trauma processing shouldn't be considered as getting stuck in the pain or having to reexperience it. I think of it as noticing the state that you're in, shifting somewhere that you prefer, and finding the meaning and connection that has always been available to you. The state of your nervous system just didn't make it safe to explore before; the protective mechanisms were too intense. Learning how to keep comfortable and connected can be quite joyful.

LET'S PRACTICE—THE BICYCLE

Another exercise I learned from Deb Dana involved imagining a bike ride.

If you don't have that much mobility or the idea is uncomfortable, any vehicle works.

Picture that the bike is coasting on a downward slope, nothing like a hill, but just a slanted road.

You can decide if you're in farm country, a coast overlooking the sea, or in the city (but don't make it busy—a bike path is best).

Let the bike speed up a bit. How does that feel in your body? (That's your movement, sympathetic system at work.)

Pump the brakes, slow things down. How does that feel? (That's your vagal brake.)

Get the bike onto a flat path. What is this feeling like now? I'm betting that's pretty easy. That's your ventral vagus feeling, smooth and calm.

CHAPTER 4

The Body Knows

When I decided to write a book about trauma, my goal was to make it much less academic than the ones that are already in existence. And while I appreciate the major book that everybody turns to, *The Body Keeps the Score*, by psychiatrist Dr. Bessel van der Kolk, it's a pretty hefty read. Especially when you've been through trauma, and your thinking brain isn't always online. It can be intimidating to pick up a few hundred scientific pages. The other renowned trauma expert Gabor Maté's insightful book *The Myth of Normal* weighs in similarly in terms of volume and academic content.

That being said, I think it's quite useful to know about the way the brain and body work. Partially because using our imagination is an incredibly powerful tool in shifting stuck patterns; it allows us to visualize the brain areas changing.

Understanding what's happening from an evolutionary perspective means that we see our reflexes as a protective mechanism. Knowing that your brain is responding just as any other animal's on the planet could decrease the shame that a person feels when trauma responses hijack their body system.

The Alarm

The one part of the body that always gets mentioned when you read or listen to anything about trauma is the amygdala. It's worth spending some time learning about these: we actually have two of them—one on either side of the brain, which has two distinct hemispheres connected by a thin bridge.

When we get input to our brain, from either the internal environment of our body or the external environment around us, anything that seems threatening goes straight to the amygdalas. When the amygdalas recognize the signal as something dangerous, they react quickly. This reaction bypasses the thinking brain.

To be self-compassionate about our trauma responses, this fact is helpful. These lower-level brain structures control most of our reactions, whether they are behavioral like running or screaming, or emotional like getting angry or fearful. They're basically reflexes.

When these amygdalas have been exposed to traumatic events, they expect more of them in the future. They become sensitive, on the lookout for threats. One of the biggest problems that happens to people is that the brain turns neutral signals into scary ones.

Sometimes, we don't consciously realize the stories we tell ourselves about how dangerous the world is, because we've carried those stories for so long. We don't always know the exact wording of these stories, but once we notice our nervous system and its patterns, the stories naturally begin to change. To heal.

The Way This Shows Up in the Brain

Maurie walks down the sidewalk with their dog on a leash. They hear the sound of a motorcycle behind them. They still have road-rash skid marks down their hip and a burn scar on their inner thigh from falling off a moped while on vacation. There was no barrier on the road; they still have nightmares about falling off a cliff. The sound of a motorcycle immediately hijacks their amygdalas. The only plausible scenarios that show up for them are the motorcycle gunning them down, their dog ending up in its path, or another tragedy. Within seconds, they grab their dog and jump into a doorway. They knock somebody over as they escape. Of course, the motorcycle stays on the road and uneventfully drives past.

The Way This Shows Up in the Body

Lin has always had a sensitive stomach; she remembers being sent home from school on the days when there was an exam. She prepares diligently, often reading under her bedcovers to study. Her anxiety seems to live in her gut. When she has a strict deadline, she hears gurgling in her stomach. She gets a bloated feeling and can't eat much food on those days. The longest she's gone without having a bowel movement was one week. But sometimes she goes twice during the night. The doctors checked her out and said there was nothing wrong; they told her it was probably an irritable bowel (IBS). They told her it's a problem with the function in the gut, so she needs to manage her anxiety better. She agrees that it correlates with times of stress, but she gets so much discomfort and bloating that it's very much a physical problem. She feels frustrated that the doctors seemed to tell her it's all in her head.

The amygdalas are the fire-fighting center of the brain. Evolutionarily, this worked out well for animals. If a leopard had to run away from a fire, the preservation instinct kicks in right away. That's obviously the *flight* response in action. If a squirrel tries to escape a bird, it might try to fend it off. That's an animal trying to *fight*. Both the flight and fight responses are part of the *sympathetic* nervous system; because your body needs to move, there needs to be active engagement. All your energy goes to your muscles, your heart, and your eyes.

If a deer is being circled by a bear, it might lie down and pretend to be dead, hoping the bear would go away. We call this the *freeze* response, or *dorsal vagal*. The energy shunts away from the muscles and the heart; everything gets limp and still. The amygdalas decide which stress response to try.

The Way This Shows Up in the World

Now, take all of those responses into the modern world. Sometimes they work; sometimes, they just make things worse.

Your boss taps you on the shoulder from behind, and your hand flies up, your coffee goes flying. That's probably not the best.

Then, your partner burns something in the toaster and the smoke detector goes off. You run out the door, down six flights of steps, and you're shaking on a bench in the park when he texts you to find out what happened.

Someone who looks like your father sits next to you at the movies. You can't concentrate on the show; it's hard to breathe. You feel stuck in the seat after the credits have rolled. While you logically know it's not your father, part of you thinks he's in disguise and following you around.

Think about trauma response as a fire station in your brain. It's constantly paying attention to the signals coming in, often amplifying them. And then, anytime it notices something that could be threatening, the fire alarm goes off.

It's playing the soundtrack related to the memory that was triggered. Loudly.

Think of how much energy it takes to be constantly vigilant. To be constantly scanning both your body and the situation around your body for anything risky.

Think of how loud it gets inside this part of your brain from all the signals coming in, with the volume dial turned up as high as it gets. And then when a fire is detected, the alarms start shrieking.

This poor distracted brain, with these alarm bells ringing all the time, imagine how hard it would be to use the rest of your mind? Pretty darn hard. Consider the brain fog, memory troubles, and inability to concentrate that happens after trauma. A lot of this is because of the rewiring in your brain around these overactive amygdalas.

But what this also means is, once you learn to notice safe things around you, those signals take a different path into your thinking brain. And over time, with skills—like the ones mentioned in the second half of this book, you will learn how to turn the volume dial down.

The amygdalas exist to protect you. The whole reason for this threat detection system is to keep you safe. Even when it's bothersome or uncomfortable, the goal is to keep you safe.

One exercise I like to do with my patients is a gratitude exercise around this exact issue. Most people have spent their life upset with how their brain works by the time they've seen me. They blame their brain for making them sad or fearful. They blame their brain for the flashbacks to memories that show up unannounced. But once we understand the purpose of all of this and realize that it's a reflex, just like pulling your hand off a hot stove, we can be more sympathetic. Being self-compassionate is a huge first step in the healing process.

LET'S PRACTICE—THE HEART

I'll invite you to try a gratitude exercise, based on a Buddhist practice from (Dr.) Sister Dang Nghiem, who writes about mindfulness after trauma:

Rub your hands together gently until you can feel a bit of warmth between them.

Place one of them over the middle of your chest, around where your heart is.

Let yourself imagine the warmth from your hand spreading into your chest.

You might imagine this warmth is showing up as light.

Pick a color that you like, blue or yellow or even sparkly.

If you're able, put your second hand behind your head, right where it connects to your neck. (If either movement isn't available, you can imagine doing it.)

You can feel the bottom of your skull, how it sits in your palm.

You might imagine the same light connecting your hand to your body here.

It's time to have a conversation between the head and the heart.

Your head wants to know what your heart is about.

My heart is about love.
All it wants is to love and to be loved.
Let your head thank your heart for caring.
Your heart wants to know what your head is about.
My head is trying to keep me safe.
All it wants is for the world to be safe.
Let your heart thank your head for wanting to protect you.

Brain Networks

There's another part of the brain I'd also like to share with you.

The word *salient* means "important or prominent"—the salience network is a region in your brain that's in charge of deciding what's important and what to pay attention to. So, it filters all the information that's bombarding your brain minute by minute. The things that you can see and experience around you, but also sensations like your body's position relative to other objects.

It's a key area of your brain related to trauma processing, but it doesn't get very much attention. Researchers have studied youth and adults who exhibit the symptoms of post-traumatic stress. When they look at their brain under a special scanner (that shows not just the structure but also the electrical activity), often functional MRI or PET scans, this is an area where changes are seen.

Changes in connection within the salience network have been linked to problems with your thinking brain in later life. So, once you've been through trauma, even though you're no longer under threat, sometimes this change in the network prevents your thinking brain from fully coming back "online." This leads to troubles with concentration and memory. It also leads to emotional shifts, either heightened or even numbed. Likewise, changes in this network can cause any of the fight, flight, or freeze symptoms well into the future.

There's another interesting area of your brain, called the default mode network (DMN), which is in charge of how you perceive yourself as an individual. Have you ever questioned how you know who you are? Wondered how your consciousness has fascinating human experiences? This is getting a little vague, but bear with me.

When researchers do studies on the brain while a person is thinking about their day, we call this *memory reconsolidation*. When your brain thinks about the past or the future, the experiences that you've been through and ones that you're anticipating, changes are observed in brain imaging. All of this has to do with your self-perception; the network that lights up on the brain scans is called the DMN.

When they've done brain scanning during experiments under the influence of certain psychedelic drugs, images showed decreased DMN activity. So, when it's said that your ego dissolves and you feel a sense of interconnectedness, that's accurate according to brain images. Because of the regions of the brain that change, you're not able to see "you" as separate anymore.

In recent research, youth exposed to trauma have fewer connections in the DMN brain regions. The way this shows up in the world is something we call an *altered sense of self*. A lot of times, a person who's been through trauma might end up with a diagnosis related to delusional thinking, because this altered sense of self can show up as *derealization*, where things just don't seem real to you. Or *depersonalization*, where you feel like your body isn't really your own. These responses make sense because the brain is trying to protect you after trauma. Altering your reality is an excellent skill when that reality is dangerous. Feeling like you're not fully in your body is very protective when your body is being harmed.

Dr. Ruth Lanius's lab in Canada does this research and continues to help our understanding of the brain after trauma. But I also want to be clear that there are some limitations to these kinds of brain-scanning tests. Many of the protocols have a small sample size, which means there are not a lot of participants. So, while we can see trends in a certain direction, it's going to take lots more research for us to understand how the brain works after trauma.

The reason these issues about the salience network and DMN are so significant for people dealing with trauma is that most available therapies are cognitive—they require your thinking brain to be online and available. But when your amygdalas take over and the reflex responses get locked in, people who've experienced trauma don't have as much access to their thought processes, or even their sense of self.

Mind or Body Doorways

Top-down therapy is using the brain to help the mind-body system. Another word for this is *cognitive* therapy—using your brain (what's on top) to alter the system. Bottom-up therapy uses the body to help the mind-body system. Another word for this is *somatic* therapy—using your body (what's on the bottom) to alter the system. From all that I've studied, I believe that the body is the best initial doorway for trauma responses. Now that you understand how the system works, it's worth exploring. So many people have said to me they've been in therapy for years but didn't get anywhere until they tried a new tactic. A new door.

One we'll open together later in the book.

CHAPTER 5

The DSM

The Psychiatric Textbook

The DSM is a strange nickname for a book about psychiatry. As mentioned earlier, its full title is *The Diagnostic and Statistical Manual of Mental Disorders*. It was produced so that the US government could track the people that they considered insane. In the early days, they were called "defective, dependent, and delinquent." I swear, I'm not joking.

I'm also, sadly, not joking when I say that homosexuality was listed as a sociopathic condition. They did not remove it from the DSM until 1984. Which matters, because when society considers being gay as a mental disorder, it propagates misunderstanding and discrimination.

Classifying "normal" ways of being as "illness" causes medical trauma. This is one way that the health-care system and the people who work in it have caused trauma to others. When it comes from a book, that would be a *systemic* or *structural trauma*. But it can come from psychiatrists and other professionals too.

In the 1970s, when the psychiatrists were convening to write the third edition of the book, the Vietnam War was winding down and the thing that was called "shell shock" during earlier conflicts was named *post-traumatic stress disorder* (PTSD). This term finally came into being because more men were being identified with trauma symptoms. It took more men experiencing trauma for academics to begin quality research on it. Just think of all the women who were called witches or hysterical when they were exhibiting mental health distress—over many centuries.

One of my primary concerns about the textbook for psychiatry is that it doesn't sufficiently recognize the importance of past and existing stressors on the symptoms that we have. What we diagnose as depression or anxiety can sometimes be a manifestation of trauma. Childhood trauma can change our brain. Social problems can cause trauma responses. We understand all of this now, based on research, but it's not reflected in the DSM-5 yet. Instead of recognizing that many of the ways people show up in the world are natural responses to their experiences, these symptoms get pathologized—so it's considered a disease, a disorder, or a deficit. Although, when you really think about it, these adaptive responses are actually strengths. They're ways that your brain and body aim to protect you.

Another significant problem with the DSM is the nonsensical separation between the brain and body. We now understand that so many of the so-called psychiatric symptoms are ways that the nervous system reacts when it's under stress. Because of the intricate connections between the brain and body, this needs to be considered when we discuss symptoms or how we try to help people.

Recent research shows that feelings are just an interpretation of physical symptoms, an expectation of the emotion that makes sense in the context. So, they manifest related to shifting perceptions within different cultures, different regions, even different generations. If you show people a photograph of various facial expressions and ask them what emotion the subject is experiencing, they'll take a guess. When the researcher changes the story behind the picture, people presume the face was showing a different emotion. They could interpret somebody whom they thought looked angry at first as anxious once the story behind the scenario is changed.

Likewise, if people are conditioned to believe that when their heart pounds, it represents fear, then that is the emotion they will interpret. By associating the racing heart with excitement, you can change this emotional experience.

LET'S PRACTICE—THE SHIFT

This practice involves noticing how your body feels, which isn't easy for everyone. If you aren't able to pay attention to these areas, figure out what is available to you. Can you notice your feet on the ground—do they feel like they want to move? Can you notice your posture and how that makes the rest of your body feel?

When you're next in a scenario that seems challenging, this is a great exercise. I'm not talking about something that's triggering or traumatizing, just a bit anxiety-provoking.

If you can, notice if your heart speeds up; you might get sweaty and clammy hands. Sometimes the stomach gets involved, twisting or getting nauseated.

Because this is a situation that might make you nervous, those physical sensations are likely going to be interpreted as fear or worry.

What if we could interpret them differently?

It's that easy. All emotions are perceptions in the brain.

Can you think about anything in the scenario that might excite you? Even if it is something stressful, we could interpret it as a welcome challenge. Can the challenge be the possibility of you feeling like you can handle it? Could that be exciting?

Could you reframe the physical sensations that you're experiencing as excitement?

The more you practice telling yourself that you're excited, the more you strengthen the pathway connecting this event or scenario to a new emotion.

Creating new neural linkages.

Look at you—changing your mind!

Diagnostic Dilemma

In early DSM days, psychiatrists diagnosed *neurosis* (what we'd now consider anxiety) in women who weren't happy as submissive housewives and gave them benzodiazepines. These medications affect our brain like alcohol—leaving these poor people in a haze.

Pharmaceutical options have increased decade by decade, linked to more DSM diagnoses that would be potentially treated with these new medications. Research funds that supported the academic careers of the psychiatrists who were involved in the books also increased. In fact, over two-thirds of the psychiatrists involved in the latest version of the DSM, the fifth edition as I write this, had ties to the pharmaceutical industry.

But don't take my word on it. Dr. Allen Frances, a psychiatrist who was heavily involved in authoring the fourth edition of DSM, wrote a book called *Saving Normal*. In it, he confirmed these ties to drug companies as being problematic. Even more important, he lamented how many new diagnostic categories were being created. He describes binge eating, where the criteria have become so loose that many of us fall into it.

Criteria that are too broad can lead to a problem of being "too sensitive." When disease criteria are too sensitive (from a scientific perspective), it means we will label too many people with it. When a disease is "too specifically" described, it means that people who have it are going to get missed. While it is arguably hard to find the perfect sweet spot—when people making decisions have ties to a profit-making industry, it would make sense that they might fall on the side of giving more patients a label—one that typically leads to a prescription.

Regarding the DSM, many researchers have been concerned about the lowered threshold to get a diagnosis of autism or attention deficit hyperactivity disorder (ADHD). The dominant paradigm of how to be considered normal is getting narrower. While I love that people who are neurodivergent can use these labels to build community and find allies, I wonder if this is another example of society pathologizing the many ways that people exist in and experience the world.

The checklist style of diagnosis isn't always encompassing of each personality and behavior. Many women are underdiagnosed with conditions like autism and ADHD. Many people present in culturally specific ways that don't fit the average checklist of how such conditions show up.

One DSM theme I've always had a problem with is the diagnosis of grief, which is considered prolonged if it's lasting for over one month. One month? Now that I've experienced it myself with family members, my best friend who passed from a brain tumor at age thirty-six, and the loss of my marriage—I know that grief is lifelong. The holes in our heart remain. No amount of medication or therapy for grief can bring a loved one back.

Another major issue with the DSM has been its lack of reliability. While there are checklists for things like depression, anxiety, and ADHD—different clinicians often have conflicting opinions on the primary diagnosis of a patient. That's an enormous problem. It discredits research that depends on having the diagnosis properly assessed (what they call *inclusion criteria* to enroll into a study trial). Ultimately, it means that many of the psychiatric diagnoses are subjective. It might be one reason that so many more women end up with one. Especially when you think of how many elderly white men created the DSM. Anything outside of their perspective might seem pathological?

Think about depression. Can we be certain that the symptoms are not related to the low-activation nervous system? Sleeping too much, no interest in things that you typically would be excited about. Feeling hopeless about the future, feeling guilty about the past. Being sad and irritable. As we just learned, these could relate to an overactive parasympathetic nervous system.

What about anxiety? Could it be a high-activation in the nervous system? Feeling restless, jittery, worried about the future. Noticing muscle tension and having difficulty sleeping. As we just learned, these could relate to an overactive sympathetic nervous system.

Many personality disorders have been linked to the ways that people learn to cope with complex trauma. Especially the diagnosis of borderline personality; "fearing abandonment" can stem from childhood neglect.

Intense relationships with a lot of rifts can result from a person reacting to loud signals of danger. Risk-taking and self-harm can be the brain's way of distracting from internal pain. And who wouldn't feel angry about going through trauma?

Narcissistic desires for attention can come from a person who had no attention as a kid when they needed it. Or even too much attention, which they interpreted as love. They might end up feeling like their self-loathing or uncertainty can be masked with the opposite.

Dependent traits would naturally result from neglect or abuse. The adult would still feel the need to seek protection and care. When I read the book about the Neuroaffective Relational Model (NARM), *Healing Developmental Trauma,* I felt the authors had a better understanding of how humans react to relational trauma than did the DSM's characterization of personality traits.

In fact, the people convening on the newest DSM decided not to include "complex trauma," as the symptoms overlapped too much with personality disorders—rather than reexamining whether these symptoms are often survival strategies.

A disturbing trend that I've noticed is how many people do the checklist for ADHD and assume they have the condition. Many of these symptoms could relate to being in an unsupportive home environment or a stressful program at school. They could relate to the tone or status of your nervous system. They could relate to the amount of coffee or alcohol that you drink. They could relate to the fact that many people just don't thrive in the way we currently set the structures of school and work. I don't want to discredit people debilitated by ADHD, but I know, just as Dr. Frances knew, there's a ton of overdiagnosis—and it's only getting worse. Young people worry about their future because of the current financial and environmental situation. Should we really be diagnosing this understandable worry as a disease? Or should we acknowledge that we have failed to keep our next generations safe?

It's also important to mention that we continue to perpetuate the disease mentality for people who don't fit gender normative rules. A person who is gender nonbinary or transgender needs to have a psychiatric diagnosis before they can pursue medications and surgical options—this is slowly changing with the most recent World Professional Association for Transgender Health (WPATH) guidelines in 2022. Rather than seeing the treatments as affirming, we view their truth as pathological. I think it's one reason there remains significant transphobia in medicine, and certainly this contributes to public opinion that harms these communities.

The DSM also maintains whiteness as being all-powerful (white supremacy). They describe non-Western phenomena as *culture-bound* (the term used by DSM to include symptoms related to cultural practices). Until the recent fifth edition, it listed these as specific syndromes. Now, there is at least an acknowledgment that culture needs to be considered. As somebody who has worked with immigrants and refugees for over twenty years, it's clear to me how the DSM upholds the white settler–colonial viewpoint.

Many of my patients who are South Asian present with physical complaints when they have anxiety or depression. I have seen arrivals from Syria or Iran who present with abdominal pain or headache, but because I have learned from these communities, I now know to ask the right questions about stress and mood. I've also learned about fascinating belief systems, such as many countries' belief in animist practices—where a person could do ill by causing bad luck and physical symptoms to befall another (like creating a spell or hex). In such scenarios, offering a medication wouldn't address their actual concern.

One final, and major, concern I have is that the DSM is tied to capitalistic structures. It examines whether a person is functional in a world that is presuming that everybody's goal is to be in a normative relationship and find traditional employment. The more time I reflect, the more I'm convinced that our life's purpose is to develop meaning and connections. I just don't see a lot of that between the pages of this particular manual.

This is my overall problem with the DSM: it doesn't acknowledge the social conditions and policies that have influenced a lot of the so-called illnesses. Were housewives in the 1960s truly suffering from neurosis, or were they lacking personal power and meaning? The Rolling Stones wrote a song about it, "running for the shelter of a mother's little helper." Are modern women suffering from skyrocketing rates of depression, or are they crushed by the responsibilities of being wives and daughters and parents and workers and volunteers, along with living up to the intimidating "perfection" they see on Instagram, all the while afraid to lose their rights over bodily autonomy? For people who use drugs to cope, what if their access to drugs is all by design for the prison industrial complex that wants to keep certain people locked up? (Many argue that modern slavery was channeled into the prison system, which keeps Black, Latinx, and Indigenous people disproportionately incarcerated.)

In the edition of the DSM that I studied, there was an opportunity to describe the factors that contributed to the disorder categories, things like social conditions and environment. Things like trauma. Considering the diagnosis of *complex trauma* didn't make it into this massive book, it seems the authors refuse to acknowledge that the root causes of many mental symptoms are often individual and systemic trauma. (Not always, but it needs to be always considered.)

THROUGH THE AGES

CHAPTER 6

Lineage

Epigenetics

When I described my immediate family along with our countries of origin, it's because ancestral trauma can be inherited.

Many years ago, I studied genetics in my undergraduate courses. Then, we learned that the body's cells contain a template of the full human genetic code, the DNA from which the 3-D body of the baby can be "printed."

We now know this was a partial truth. *Epigenetics* flipped what we thought we knew on its head.

The best way I can explain epigenetics is that the "brain" of the cell isn't where we thought it was. The nucleus is the part of the cell where the genetic code lives. I was always taught that this was the "brain." But it's the interaction of the cell with the outside environment that decides which parts of the code turn on and get activated. So, ultimately, the cell wall is the "brain."

It makes perfect sense to me. We now understand more about the kinds of damage environmental toxins can do to your immune and nervous systems. Not to mention certain kinds of neurochemicals in your bloodstream—the kinds that show up when you're stressed out, mainly cortisol and adrenaline. Exposing your cells to these things, they turn on more illness codes. It's why certain conditions, like type 1 diabetes or fibromyalgia, often show up after a stressful event—including a viral illness. I'm sure we're going to learn lots more about the impact of stress on our cells with more research into long COVID.

There has been a lot of research into epigenetics. It shows us how intergenerational trauma, which is inherited, is encoded in the DNA that's passed down from parents to children. For example, researchers exposed mice in a lab to a smell and simultaneously provided an uncomfortable mild shock. This association of discomfort to the smell resulted in mice actively avoiding the smell. This avoidance was passed down to (at least) the next two generations of mice.

Research has demonstrated the mechanism of how this takes place. They studied it in Holocaust survivors; their DNA had new codes, based on this horrifying experience. These changes were handed down, permanently altering the lineage.

After the Twin Towers fell on 9/11, pregnant women at late stages who developed PTSD passed the trauma responses to their children—a study showed their babies had higher levels of stress hormones in their saliva.

So, if you think about true healing of trauma, it's not just your own that you should be examining. Sometimes traumatic responses like avoidance or fear don't come from our personal experience; they're something we were born with.

There might be a person who's afraid of thunder and lightning. Is it possible that an ancient ancestor had a traumatic event related to lightning or fire?

Imagine a person who is afraid of people in uniform. They've never had an unpleasant experience with an authority figure that they can remember. But perhaps their great-grandfather might have been in the army or been harmed by invading people during a war.

Imagine a person who can't seem to trust their partner in a relationship. Although nobody cheated on them, this might have happened to their mother or grandmother. It's harder for them to resolve, because they're not even certain what the original trauma looked like. It might feel impossible to process when there's no actual memory to deal with; just a felt sense that certain situations don't feel safe.

Fawning

At the risk of recommending too many books, I'm going to give a shout-out to one by Mark Wolynn, titled *It Didn't Start with You.* Part of the reason I'm writing this book is because I've read hundreds of books about trauma. I have the time, energy, and privilege to have done it. Some of those books are quite academic, with complicated terms and an expectation of medical understanding. So, here, I'm distilling the ideas.

Here is an idea from Dr. Wolynn: *We may attract friends, partners, or colleagues who do the same behaviors we reject in our family.*

This pattern can cause the *fawn* response, often seen after trauma. It looks like people-pleasing. This tends to be a person influenced by their inner child who believes if they were just "good enough," they'd get the love they seek. The rejection doesn't have to be in conscious memory—if a child is separated from their mom before the age of three, that gets held in their nervous system as abandonment and distress. Finding the love you yearn for can help you let go of wanting love from someone who was (and may remain) unavailable. Sometimes this looks like *rejection sensitivity*—someone who is assuming they're going to be rejected even without the evidence.

Another common defense strategy is to push people away. People with rejection sensitivity might do that to avoid rejection.

Personal journaling is often done to explore your own experiences, but sometimes it's helpful to imagine the ones that might have happened before your generation. Especially if there are still people to ask or sources where you can search for more information. An understanding of where some of your own limiting beliefs might have originated can help you work through them yourself.

Here's an Example

Selena always thought that her mom hated her. She never felt a lot of warmth from her and gravitated more to her father. Even though, technically, there was no abuse, there just wasn't a strong connection. When Selena started seeing a therapist, questions showed up about her family background and she asked her mom for the first time. She learned her grandmother had escaped El Salvador after the murder of her husband. Circumstances separated her only son from her on the journey and she never learned how he disappeared or if he was alive. She made it to America pregnant and alone. That sense of fear and horror lived in her bloodstream and was passed to her baby. So, when Selena's mother was born, she was already in a soup of stress chemicals.

Once Selena started examining this story with her therapist, they came to understand that her mom was dissociative. She distracted herself with work and housework to avoid feeling her emotions. She was also deathly afraid of poverty, anything that would put her family at risk. So, she worked three jobs while Selena was growing up to ensure their financial stability. While Selena had a roof over her head, she didn't have the cuddles and storytelling that would have provided a deeper sense of security.

Selena learned that it wasn't her mom's fault. She wrote her a letter and symbolically mailed it to their old address in El Salvador. Once the therapist got deeper into the history, they recognized nobody had processed the loss of her grandfather and uncle, because they were immigrants struggling to survive. So, Selena designed a process to commemorate their lives. She learned that her uncle had been a guitar player, something she had always been interested in, and she learned how to play. Over time, writing songs became something that helped her release stress and tension. Music came easily to her; melodies would show up in her head. She imagined it was a gift from her uncle, which brought her peace. Her mother always loved the songs, which gave them a language where they could share feelings.

Our Ancestors

Healing the trauma of our lineage is impactful work. It's one way that human consciousness evolves and expands. So many of our ancestors were in survival mode, dealing with wars and migration, racism, and intense poverty. Many of us couldn't imagine the conditions that our ancestors lived in one hundred years ago, never mind three hundred or beyond.

Even if you know little about your family history, it's equally important to work with feelings and sensations. Your body remembers.

Although there is hidden trauma in our ancestral backgrounds, there is also great strength. It's important when we deal with trauma to take an asset-based approach. There were vulnerabilities, but our ancestors survived to give birth to another human, centuries ago when maximum life expectancy was only thirty or forty years—it's almost miraculous. It means that the humans from which we are descended were true warriors. This is something we can use as a tool for our own healing.

LET'S PRACTICE—THE TREE

This is a guided imagery exercise. I attached a longer version of it to the QR code (see page xviii) that links you to the Modern Trauma website.

Sit with your back against a chair with both of your feet touching the ground, if you are able. If you aren't, try to focus on the parts of your body that are touching a chair or bed, wheelchair, or the ground.

Begin by taking some deep breaths. You might focus on the inhale or the exhale if that feels good for your body. Deeper inhalations give you more energy, longer exhalations release stress.

Begin with the part of your body that is closest to the ground and flat against it. That's probably the soles of your feet. Imagine that they are sprouting roots. It might start off as short tendrils, but eventually, they get longer and thicker. They start to look like gnarled tree roots, the kind that displaces the sidewalk. These are deep underground. At least four feet.

Now imagine that your body is the trunk of this tree. Your core is the main part, solid and substantial. The energy from the roots feeds this part of the tree, but it has its own power and sturdy strength.

Visualize the energy flowing from the roots up into the trunk. I like to imagine this as representing the inner energies of the earth: lava that's a thick, fiery liquid. This powerful fire can flow through the roots and up into your entire body.

Send this energy wherever it needs to go.

With every breath, imagine the pulse of the energy spreading its warmth and vitality throughout the entire system.

You might imagine that your arms are branches and your fingers are leaves.

It's always beautiful to imagine leaves. What color would they be? Would you be able to see through them on a sunny day? Imagine looking at the delicate veins that are infused with the earth's energy.

Can you imagine the animals that are sheltered underneath or within this tree? Are there mushrooms growing from the trunk? Can you hear the buzzing of bees? Any nests in the branches? This tree is intimately connected to the web of life.

It's also deeply connected to all of the other ancestors. The roots that travel into the earth also shoot sideways, so all trees in the forest are interconnected. These linkages provide communication and support. They warn of danger. They send healing energy when needed.

Now, imagine the beauty of the surrounding forest. You are not a tree lonely on the top of a hill. You're surrounded by these other living beings, each one connected to the earth's energy—just like you.

Decolonized Exploration

The concept of ancestors is one that is held in deep reverence by Indigenous people on the land where I live and study. While I'm not an expert on *neurodecolonization*, I have attended seminars with some thought leaders, so I understand that this broadly refers to the decolonizing (bringing forth Indigenous ways of being) of our mind. Indigenous scholars have a lot to contribute when it comes to ancestral healing. Their core idea that every decision needs to consider seven generations behind and seven generations ahead is one that would solve a lot of trauma caused by oppressive systems. The books *Decolonizing Trauma Work* and *Decolonizing Methodologies* (about research) helped me form these thoughts, and I'd recommend exploring these and connect with Indigenous academics in your region.

First, I would like to focus on the idea of *family*. While I don't have children of my own, I have chosen some of my family. I met Aishwarya while she was in her undergraduate training and now consider her like a daughter, while respecting the relationship she has with her parents. I believe in the concept of a *chosen family*; so many people are not cherished within biological family units and so they seek relationship with others. Or they may find a person who belongs in their heart, without a formal relationship like "sister" or "partner." Aishwarya's mother, Geeta, says our relationship is *karma*, which is a beautiful thought about being destined.

I studied a course in adolescent psychology from an Indigenous lens with Dr. Martin Brokenleg. He told us that the Lakota (a Native American tribe) word for family encompasses about three hundred people spread out over five generations. Imagine if we could look after one another in these ways. Social isolation and loneliness would not be so pervasive.

I once listened to a lecture by Dr. Michael Yellowbird, a professor of sociology. The most impactful analogy I'd heard in a long time was when he described modern humans as wanting to be on the top of a mountain, always striving and achieving from the framework of capitalism. But an Indigenous way would be to become one with the mountain, to recognize our interconnectedness. Part of Dr. Yellowbird's work is reclaiming the wisdom that previous generations of Indigenous elders held around healing. Dancing, song, connecting to the spirit of the earth—these traditions were sacred and transformative to the original peoples of this land. And they are also part of what we, as modern people making our way in this confusing society, might be subconsciously missing.

Both Dr. Yellowbird and Dr. Brokenleg speak of the shifting of culture. What we have valued in modern society is productivity and technological accomplishments. Art and creativity, relationships, and stewarding our connection to nature have not been deemed valuable. I believe that there is an ongoing resurrection of these priorities.

I don't want to fetishize Indigenous knowledge, especially ideas that are not mine, but I believe that many other cultures had similar ways of knowing. When I was visiting colleagues in Vancouver for a weekend forum on Indigenous healing, one of my favorite exercises was being led through a series of *circle dances* from around the world. We all formed a circle and performed intricate rhythms of patterns, all moving as one. I wasn't just moved physically. Being part of a collective body, embodying that synergy, is very special. I even learned a dance that was Celtic from my background. There are many from Eastern Europe as well. Perhaps my Ukrainian ancestors also did one. Very few of us have a strong connection to our ancestors in this way.

Dr. Daniel Foor wrote a book and offered an online course on "Ancestral Medicine." He teaches people to find out as much as we can about our lineage and how to communicate with ancestors, who can guide and teach us and whom we can forgive. He cautions against contacting those who are not yet well (still struggling with their own unresolved traumas). In his book, he mentions that many cultures continue a relationship with ancestors who have passed away: including the Celtic Samhain, Mexico's Día de los Muertos (Day of the Dead), and Japan's Obon Festival.

Here's an Example

Many cultures have small shrines in the yard or home to respect their ancestors. I worked for many months in Laos in eastern Asia, where these shrines are commonplace. They're often tall, red wooden structures with offerings in silver bowls of rice and oranges. People tied on white and saffron bracelets to represent connections among the living and the spiritual worlds. I was fortunate to be included in such ceremonies (*baci*), once being invited to become a member of my friend's village. I will never forget the feeling of having dozens of people tying a bracelet around my wrist and making a wish for my future.

In my house in Canada, after my dad and grandma passed away, I created a space where I feel the most connected to them. A watch from each.

Photographs of them, youthful and at peace. Plus other personal items that have meaning for me.

If you were to have a connection to your ancestors, those who held ancient traditions, what would that look like? How could you find out more? What would you like to offer them—foods, flowers, stones, herbs, or seeds? Would you light a candle?

Is there music that connects you to your heritage? Would it be meaningful for you to play a traditional song that has been sung for centuries? Not only can this be powerful without being translated (certain Celtic and Ukrainian songs bring me to tears), it gives these ancestors ongoing life in keeping the music alive in modern times.

Developing a relationship with your ancestry is often possible, even if your immediate family doesn't feel safe. Understanding how trauma passes through generations can create compassion for yourself and others in your family.

CHAPTER 7

Preverbal

While trauma manifests in people through similar body responses, there are two separate pathways to get there.

If you experience events where your body (or someone you love) is at risk, that's the *shock trauma pathway*. You believe that the world isn't safe. In this scenario, exposure to fearful experiences while being in a calm body will be part of the healing process.

If you experienced adults who were supposed to be caregivers but not able to be consistent or safe, this is an *attachment trauma*. You believe that people aren't safe. In this scenario, exposures to trusting relationships while being in a calm body will be part of the healing process.

So, you can see that the calm body figures into both of these paths. We will spend a lot of time on that in the second half of this book. Complex trauma tends to involve both paths.

Pregnancy

When I was a family doctor, women (also trans men and folks who don't identify as women but have a uterus) who became pregnant for the second time sometimes said that they couldn't recall the first birth. During the few times I had been involved in the delivery of a baby, it looked messy and painful. Yet, think about how many centuries of childbirth took place without modern interventions like painkillers and surgery. Although those are some reasons why maternal mortality rates have improved so much.

It makes sense that, if something goes wrong, childbirth would be incredibly traumatic. The fear of having something happen to a newborn is terrifying, especially because it's such a complicated procedure. If the baby is stressed, it has a poop inside the womb. This debris, called *meconium*, is dangerous for the baby to inhale into their lungs (they don't breathe before birth, as they get nutrients through the umbilical cord).

It's estimated that one-third of mothers who experience a complicated delivery of their baby could have a formal diagnosis of PTSD.

I've also seen mental health issues in women who didn't experience compassion from the hospital staff during this time. Many immigrants and refugees don't speak the local language fluently, so when they're being given instructions during childbirth, they can't always comply. We often ignore their cultural practices and hopes for the delivery. While there is a push to have more cultural sensitivity in these environments, we still have a long way to go. Imagine the feeling of powerlessness a pregnant person has when giving birth while lacking communication and appropriate support.

The fears that develop at such a pivotal transition in a person's life can get locked in. Risk factors include an emergency delivery like a C-section (surgery), using instruments like vacuums and forceps to help the baby come out, or a susceptible mom because of past experiences. This trauma might show up as a parent who can't let their baby out of their sight. This would correlate to the hypervigilance of the high-activation stress response (the sympathetic nervous system). It could also show up as a parent who feels disconnected from their child, more in keeping with avoidance related to a low-activation stress response (the dorsal vagal system). The latter often gets diagnosed as postpartum depression—which is a common phenomenon too.

About one-quarter of new mothers have at least one symptom of PTSD. It's probably much more common than we realize because, like many women's health issues, there simply isn't enough research. This is compounded because women who are afflicted may be embarrassed. They would feel like it's not normal for them to have nightmares about the birth, something that was supposed to be positive and joyful.

Imagine the pain of your own child being a trigger. Your own baby brings back the pain from their birth experience. Fears that continue to live in your body.

Babes

Now, let's look at the whole scenario from the child's perspective. Since newborns don't have an easy way of communicating, we must rely on what we know about biology and our observations.

Inside the uterus, where a clump of cells grows into an infant, it is like being immersed in a bath. There's warm amniotic fluid where you're floating; everything feels like a cushion. Toward the end, you would probably feel constricted because your entire body is pushing on the walls inside the uterus. This is the only environment you've ever known. You've listened to the voice of your mother interacting all day—maybe you heard her sing. The voice of your father, if he's around, would be fuzzier, but probably recognizable. (Of course, these are the traditional versions of the family and it's important to recognize the diversity of birthing parents, and many families will have parents of the same gender.)

Certain hormones create a bond between mother and child prior to delivery. While there's an obvious physical bond, part of that bond is chemical. *Oxytocin* is a hormone that's involved in the connection between birth parents and child. Levels of this chemical peak during the labor process. Studies of the hormone have found that it's related to connection and empathy. So, it shouldn't be a surprise that it's also involved when a baby is breastfed, contributing to the bonding process. When you have enough oxytocin, it's very relaxing. Notably, the baby also produces oxytocin during childbirth. Unfortunately, being stressed during labor will lower the levels of oxytocin and increase the hormones related to stress for both mother and baby.

Picture being a baby whose home forcefully pushes them out. The muscular walls of the house that you've known for your entire existence compress around you in an unpredictable repeating pattern. The movement propels you into a tunnel that doesn't seem big enough to accommodate your size. A baby doesn't have a cognitive thought process, but I would imagine the sensation of being pushed through a hole that's clearly not big enough must feel uncomfortable. Typically, the hole widens enough that you can get through. Sometimes it doesn't. In that scenario, you would be born with somebody slicing into the wall of the snug home that you're connected to.

Either way, your first experience of the world is to go from a dark, warm, fluid setting to a bright, colder, less connected experience. You immediately have to figure out how to breathe air, you hear louder sounds through air instead of fluid, and you're suddenly being touched and cradled by foreign hands checking on your health status. It's no wonder that the first thing that we often notice is the newborn baby crying—imagine the stress of that shock! Something cold touches your chest to listen, they poke your heel for a blood test, and suddenly you must eat by swallowing instead of having nutrients flow through your umbilical cord. That's a lot of stress all at once.

Every human goes through it. All mammals do. Think of special circumstances like twin pregnancy, when the sibling that shares your tiny home becomes a separate body.

There's research around adoption trauma that shows that babies going to loving homes still experience separation anxiety from the birth parents. Adopted kids have increased diagnoses of mental illness and substance use. Even with a kind family, even with an open adoption keeping contact with birth parents, even when everything goes right—a trauma has still occurred. As we've seen in other mammals, they know their mother by scent. So, from the first day of separation, the familiar smell is missing. The babies subconsciously feel abandoned, even betrayed.

Many issues can stem from this very early loss—lack of trust, sense of rejection, not feeling "good enough," uncertainty and confusion, and not having control. The baby will mourn the separation without knowing the language of grief.

Many times, the child copes with this by letting the nervous system take over. At these early stages, with no conscious thought, stress would naturally show up in behaviors. The *fight-or-flight response* would look like an infant who is irritable and fussy, crying all the time, or pushing things away that come near. Their subconscious thoughts might develop into being afraid that the world isn't a consistent place, where everything you know has become completely disrupted. The *freeze response* would look passive, disinterested, and disconnected. Their subconscious thoughts might develop into a fear of love, knowing that it might not stick around.

Separation trauma is the distrust in the world that is felt immediately and then throughout the child's life. In order to adapt, the child has to become observant to figure out how to become a member of this new family. Relying on a new person or people to meet its needs, the adopted child might become a people-pleaser who tries to always be perfect to be accepted. Or they might accept their grief and have a constant sense that something is always missing or wrong.

Here's an Example

Ana's birth mother didn't get prenatal care. She presented to the hospital in later stages of labor, while in active withdrawal from fentanyl (a potent drug related to heroin). Child protective services was called as soon as she was in the emergency room. They did not give her birth mother any painkillers during the labor, as the health-care workers decided it might interfere with whatever she had in her system already (though she was in withdrawal and could have tolerated them).

Ana went straight to the neonatal intensive care unit for high-risk babies and put on formula. Police arrested her mother for drug possession. Ana went through fentanyl withdrawal as a baby in the hospital, shivering and sweating through her first lonely days. The bright lights of the incubator and the rubbery touch of gloves would have been her only contact with the outside world.

Because there was no plan for the baby, Ana entered protective services and shuffled through five foster homes before the age of two. Everybody thought she was developmentally slow because she wasn't speaking by then. Her world was so confusing and overstimulating, she was already dissociating.

Foundations

Think of how often, when we are unbelievably sad, we curl up into the fetal position. The position that we would have held before life became complicated. When our needs were met. Or at least, they should have been.

Think of how often those needs may not have been met before you had language to understand what that meant. This preverbal time shapes our foundational beliefs about our world. So, it's very hard for us to do talk therapy, what we called top-down, when these beliefs form before we had the language to understand them.

As adults, we try to make meaning out of our sensations, and so we create words and stories for those feelings. For some people, these beliefs don't exist in words, just in feelings. These might be more accessible to us, and possible to shift through body sensations.

One tool that sociologist Brené Brown describes is to remind yourself that your thoughts are stories. She says, "What is the story you're telling yourself?" when she thinks about a scenario—an example might be your friend cancels a plan, and your story is that she's angry (which seems likely if your parents always seemed tense when you were young). Or if a partner forgets your birthday, and the story that shows up to explain why is that they don't care about you (if your parents didn't meet your physical and emotional needs). If you think of your thoughts as stories, you can find an alternative story that could also be true.

LET'S PRACTICE—THE FOUNDATIONS

Think of a foundational belief that you have, one that shapes the way you interact. I'll give you some examples to get started:

> *The world is unsafe.*
> *Bad things happen to me.*
> *Everything is a struggle.*
> *I don't feel connected to others.*
> *Nobody cares about me.*
> *Everything is hopeless.*
> *I don't have the power to make any changes.*

Now, consider what you know about your childhood before you had language, what kinds of scenarios might have contributed to this foundational belief.

What might we do to reassure this inner child that the opposite statement could be possible? Imagine yourself as an infant, small and vulnerable. Imagine holding yourself as a child in your arms, gently rocking them and murmuring reassuring phrases.

This is reparenting.

Neurons

The neural networks that shape our brain as adults form very early. The pathways that are created in a baby's mind are incredibly fast, the most growth that we'll ever have in our lives.

Our first experiences, environments, and connections lay the framework for how we see the world and our relationships in it. While they might not feel logical as adults, and our rational mind knows they aren't true, once the preverbal mind has these fixed beliefs, it can be quite hard to shift them.

An early belief isn't just a thought—it's a foundation laid in our subconscious structures. Because we hold these preverbal beliefs in the centers of our mind without language, I don't advocate for talk therapy as the first step, or the only step, in healing from early childhood trauma.

In fact, the best languages of the preverbal mind are imagery and metaphor. I use a lot of interactive guided imagery through my practice. Imagining a tree and its roots when you think about your ancestors is one example of using these skills.

Let's do another quick exercise using these powerful tools that interact with our subconscious mind.

BOUNDARIED

We begin forming boundaries at this preverbal stage.

This word is subjective, but here's my interpretation: *Boundaries are the ways that we set the expectations of how we will be treated.*

Imagine a small baby who feels their care is an imposition. This child may grow up to feel that they should accept whatever boundary is forced on them.

What about one who senses that they are being held too closely by a parent who's suffering from depression? In that case, this smothering feeling might make them create strict boundaries with this parent or others in the future.

Now, imagine a small child who doesn't have any sense of care from their parents. No one attends to their cries, meets their reach, or mirrors their facial expression. This child might be clingy and inappropriately chasing relationships. In therapy terms, this behavior in adulthood is called *co-dependency.* (As you know, I don't love labels. I'd rather figure out the root causes of these issues.)

In these scenarios, each child would form boundaries at a time where they didn't have the language to understand the need. They would only know that the creation of boundaries helps them feel safe. When examining why this might be as an adult, rather than language, it's simply a *felt sense.*

This is why it's useful to use imagery and metaphor to shift these early beliefs.

LET'S PRACTICE—BOUNDARIES

Take an object that reminds you of the person with whom you are working on a boundary. It could be an item of their clothing, a gift that they gave you, or something that just makes you think of them. A color or texture of fabric. Anything at all to represent them in your mind.

Place the object about one foot in front of you from where you're sitting. Look at it and imagine that this person is sitting quite close. Pay attention to what shows up in your body. Does your heart pound a little faster? If you aren't connected to your inner sensations, what emotions do you notice? Do you feel you want to push the object away?

Let's do that. Push the object to the other side of the room. As far as it can get without losing sight of it all together. With the object so much farther, how do you feel now? Is there a part of you that wants to pick it up? Is there a part of you that wants to kick it further? You can do either of those things, then check in again with how your body feels after.

Now, pick up the object and place it in your lap. This gives you almost no boundary with what represents this person. Are you comfortable with this? With them right on top of you? How does any discomfort show up in your body? Your emotions?

Next, place the object at a distance that feels comfortable right now. Where could it be in order for your body to feel calm?

Think back to the person who you were representing with the object. How are you able to maintain the distance with them that makes you feel safest? What do you do when they get too close? What do you do when they feel too far? How can you tell inside your body, in your thought processes and in your interactions, when the boundary feels good?

Our Internal Family

We form our first feelings about the safety of the world at very young ages. One of the interesting experiences I've had with non-Western medicine (hypnotherapy or plant journeys) is the ability to tap into my memories of these very young ages. I've been able to reexperience the world through those innocent eyes.

Another therapy modality that helps us access these younger parts is Internal Family Systems (IFS), developed by a psychologist named Dr. Dick Schwartz. He speaks of some of these younger parts that encountered serious challenges as the Exiles. Your integrated, clear, and compassionate Self can soothe these Exiles. Sometimes, this technique uses imagery, where you might imagine taking the young child in your lap and holding them. Sometimes, it's a dialogue, where you have a conversation explaining to them the truth of what you now know. "Right here, right now, we are safe," "You will survive this," or "We got out."

It's important to know that we can access these parts of us that hold foundational beliefs. We can re-create early experiences and shift our preverbal feelings.

Reparenting

One amazing experience that I had, just before the COVID-19 pandemic hit, was at the Esalen Institute on the rugged coast in California. This place hosted the Beat poets of the sixties, and some of the earliest trauma work happened here. I joined a weeklong retreat to study with Dr. Bessel van der Kolk (author of *The Body Keeps the Score*).

The retreat started with a lot of PowerPoint slides about his research and ideas around trauma. I'd already done a yearlong program through his institute, the Trauma Research Foundation, so these were mostly familiar to me.

What I didn't know was that he was preparing us for the last two days together. He was getting to know the audience, through our questions and the sessions where we did movement or song with his wife, Licia Sky. Then, he chose some participants to enact something he calls *psychodrama*. This is when a person moves to the center of a circle, choosing from the others in the group to represent their real and their ideal parents. The ideal parents hold them and say kind words, in a powerful reparenting exercise.

Healing these foundational beliefs might take creativity. But it can be done.

When children don't have attuned parents who help them learn to self-soothe, this often shows up as soothing in unusual (like stimming [repetitive movements] or hyperfocus) or dangerous (like risk-taking or substance use) ways as adults. But when we have safe people in our lives, we can learn to attune to them and shift these habits when we model their behavior.

Humanity is the culmination of generations of parents who try to survive, to keep their families safe, and to learn on their journey through life. There's great power in acknowledging all of this, so that we can create better conditions for parents and newborns to thrive.

CHAPTER 8

Growing Up Aces

The Study

Once a baby learns to speak, to walk, and to do more tasks—they will remember their experiences. The brains of children develop at a fast and complex rate. New neurons create the foundation of their belief system for the rest of their lives. If they encounter trauma at this critical age, it becomes a part of that foundation—like holes in the concrete of a home.

A study was done in the 1990s where a large medical organization in Southern California examined childhood trauma. The results of this research project, titled Adverse Childhood Experiences (ACE), should have changed everything in medical education and health care.

The research started when Dr. Vincent Felitti worked at a weight-loss clinic. He noticed that almost all the patients with significant obesity could lose weight for a short amount of time, but it often came back. One person finally said to him that she felt like it protected her. When he asked about childhood abuse, he realized that for many of these patients, they considered the weight a physical barrier to help them stay safe.

These conversations got the doctor curious. He asked the organization if he could do a study, and they ended up sending surveys to seventeen thousand people. And what they found was shocking.

They discovered the rates of childhood trauma were much higher than anybody could have ever predicted. But more important than that, for every trauma that the adult remembered experiencing, there was an exponential rise in the medical problems they had later in life.

Exponential in a way that we'd never seen before. With every additional trauma on the survey (scored out of ten), both physical and psychiatric illnesses rise sharply. For a score of zero, people had few health problems. But if they had one or two of the experiences that the survey asked about, they had obvious health problems. And people who had six or more? Literally, their lives were shorter.

I don't want to get too far into the details of this study, because I promised you a book that wasn't too academic. But what we understand about childhood trauma because of this research is important. And the survey that they used has now turned into the ACE questionnaire, which is something that health clinics may use to find out the history from their clients. Unfortunately, the questionnaire wasn't intended to be used in this way. Because they designed it for a study, it's more of a public health tool to uncover population-level responses rather than giving a doctor specific information about their patient.

It seems we've jumped straight into childhood trauma here. So, let's persist for a bit before we widen the lens.

Ten Questions

Here is the list of the ten questions that are on the ACE survey:

Abuse—emotional, physical, or sexual

Neglect—emotional or physical

Household Challenges—violence toward mother, substance use in the house, mental illness in the house, parents who separated, or somebody went to prison

Check In

I didn't put a trigger warning in this chapter, because you've picked up a book about trauma and so you probably expected there to be some challenging content.

One reason I'm hesitant to use the ACE questionnaire is because it can be unsettling. To find out not just that your score is on the higher end of the ten, but to find out what it means from a public health perspective.

Please note that, no matter what the research shows, your story is your story. In fact, there are positive childhood and adult experiences that can shift the balance again.

You are managing your trauma—right now. And hopefully with a trained professional, if that's available to you. By learning to shift your nervous system, this may help you avoid any potentially bad outcomes—this is under investigation. While the original research didn't go into the physiological reasons trauma has these implications later in life, we can easily speculate.

When you're in a sympathetic nervous system response, your body sends energy to the heart and muscles. It actively turns off your immune system. This makes you more susceptible to infections and autoimmune disease and blocks cellular self-repair. Likewise, once you learn how to unlock from the fight-or-flight response, your immune system returns to full functioning.

Another factor is that people who've experienced these kinds of trauma sometimes need to dissociate or distract (with drugs, alcohol, or smoking), which might put them at higher risk for lung disease or cancer.

With the people at the weight-loss clinic, food was part of their coping strategy. It's one that many humans share, including me. But this method of coping comes at a price, from high cholesterol or blood pressure to inflammation in blood vessels and organs. These factors can lead to a host of other medical problems.

It's clear that trauma causes mental and physical health issues—this entire book makes that connection.

Looking at the ACE survey can bring up many emotions. Let's take a minute to acknowledge these and identify what has shown up. Check in to see if you have any physical symptoms.

And now, please remind yourself with your cognitive brain that you are doing the work. You are on the journey toward healing. As you spend less

ADVERSE & POSITIVE CHILDHOOD EXPERIENCES

INDIGENOUS AND LINEAGE WISDOM

ECOSYSTEM

Fire damage

Pollution & poisoning

Natural disasters

Species under threat

Climate crisis

Ocean & land instability

Divorce

Neglect

Abuse

FAMILY

Illness

Addictions

Bullying

Parental care

Serve-and-return interactions

Listening & connection

Support

Nature

Housing or food insecurity

Strong relationships

Healthy brain and body

COMMUNITY CARE

Ritual & tradition

Sports & activities

Open conversations

Safe spaces

Belonging

Art & creativity

Chosen family

Mental health supports

COLLECTIVE

Poverty

Bullying

Structural violence

Food scarcity

Violence

Classism

Attacks on race, gender, sexuality, age

Ancestral trauma

Suppressed opportunities

Discrimination

Credit: PACES Connection, ACEs Connect, Nadine Burke-Harris, Donna Jackson Nakazawa

time in the activated nervous system, your natural immune system and repair will engage.

Limitations

It's important also to recognize the limitations of the ACE survey. It mentions a parent that goes to prison or divorce but not one that dies while you're growing up. I don't know why the researchers left "death of a parent" off their questionnaire—perhaps because it's uncommon—but this proves it's not meant as a comprehensive screening test.

A racialized person might experience microaggressions at school, have fears of police violence, or face overt racism in a way that other kids would never encounter. All of this can create a trauma response.

Or somebody who grows up in an unsafe neighborhood, where there are unpredictable threats and crimes—that could also lead to hypervigilance and anxiety. When you believe the world isn't safe, and you have evidence that this is the case, it sets up extra-strong foundational beliefs.

Something I encountered a fair bit growing up was bullying. And I believe it's much worse for kids growing up today, because there are so many new ways to do it online. When I was bullied, it was being mocked on the playground or pushed around on the school bus. It was having my friends turn on me when they decided that associating with me could be a social liability. Those things hurt, don't get me wrong. But the level of bullying that takes place over social media is different. The kinds of things that are said are so much more harmful and violent than anything I encountered.

Dr. Nadine Burke Harris is a pediatrician and advocate who uses a longer ACE questionnaire that includes more items in it (you can read about it in her book *The Deepest Well*). She also creates programming to help parents keep a calm home environment, as well as mental health support for kids. If only this kind of preventative, focused care were available everywhere.

Risk Taking

There have always been kids with self-destructive tendencies. What I didn't understand, until I read a book by Dr. Janina Fisher about trauma survivors, is that these are coping strategies. People aren't trying to be destructive; these strategies are trying to help.

When a child faces neglect or abuse, they start to believe that they don't matter, and their future looks hopeless. In that scenario, it's easy to feel indifferent about safety. Self-harm, thinking about not being alive, eating disorders, and substance use tend to have their origins between the ages of ten and fourteen.

But the cause happens long before that. Their behaviors are trying to seek relief from physical and emotional pain. It's hard to imagine how this soothes, but it's easy to see how it distracts. Or it could confirm the fact that the brain is already sending signals that the world is dangerous. It's familiar, the world makes sense—this is *congruence*.

If a child has experienced a lot of abuse or neglect, safe and calm sensations and emotions are sometimes experienced as threatening. It's not familiar. Their brain wonders when the next shoe will drop.

Harmful behaviors can mean that there's a part of us that can't handle the constant internal pain and needs to create new sensations.

From a biology perspective, a lot of these behaviors start adrenaline production. This can give you a burst of energy and a feeling of control—just when you need both. When your stress hormones (like cortisol) are active in your body, it also works like an anesthetic (the drugs that help you fall asleep before surgery). When a stress is happening, your body shuts down some of the pain receptors so that you can push through the stressor no matter what kind of injury you have. You can see how this would be adaptive through evolution. If something is chasing you and you sprain your ankle, you don't want to slow down to tend to it. So, if the stress hormones turn down the signals of pain, this helps you escape. This anesthetic (including anti-inflammatory) effect can temporarily help with lowering the pain signals from physical sensations or emotions.

It's less shameful to situate these destructive behaviors in the context of self-protection. One of the terrible things that these ACE traumas do to a child is make them feel like they weren't deserving of love and care. If your own parents harmed you, or didn't protect you from threat, you believe that you deserve bad things to happen to you. This shame becomes internalized. It's one of the hardest things for me to deal with in treating complex trauma.

LET'S PRACTICE—THE LITTLES

Picture yourself as a child dealing with something stressful. Don't think of a trauma listed in the survey; we want to start small because if you create success with these exercises, your body learns how to stay calm even when remembering challenging experiences. Think back to an accident where you had a minor injury, mild difficulty at school, an irritating interaction while shopping, or losing an object of significance. Something that was frustrating or annoying, but not more difficult than that.

Let's name the feeling you would have had at the time. When I was a kid, I was obsessed with a British series of square books with simple characters in them that had silly little adventures. They were called Little Miss and Little Mister. Mr. Messy was my favorite, for obvious reasons. You don't have to label yours with any kind of gender, but you could imagine a name that suits the emotion attached to the memory. Frustrated Felix. Irritated Izzy. Upset Unicorn. Once you've given it a name, and it seems cute, you might consider drawing it—if that's in your tool kit and you have the materials handy. I like to use Sharpies; there's something so pleasing about the bright colors.

Ask your little character what they're worried about. You might draw it as a speech bubble. Always use the language of *them*, that *they* are feeling a certain way. Part of healing is to leave the past in the past, to stop identifying with the emotions that were being felt.

Next, ask them what they need to hear to feel reassured. If you've imagined the little being, add whatever it is they need to your mental imagery. If you drew them, see if you can make the situation better for them in the drawing.

Now, check in with your body. How did that exercise feel? Did it give you some distance from the original event?

Teenage Brain

Dr. Dan Siegel is a psychiatrist who speaks a lot about the adolescent brain. He describes that this is a time of intense growth of the neural network, as well as the best time to specialize areas of the brain where there's talent or interest. Rather than thinking of this time as a challenge, he sees it as an opportunity.

Part of the opportunity is how we find community. It's evolution. All animals venture away from their parents and start seeking a peer group in the time of adolescence. It's a group that infers protection and support. It's very difficult for humans when we can't find our peers. Anything that makes us feel different, anything that makes us feel like we don't fit in, is incredibly hard during this time. It's simple biology.

Many people with an adolescent brain, before the age of twenty-five, feel isolated and alone. They feel that it's very difficult to find people who they resonate with, where they might belong.

When a teenager says to their parent that they want a certain pair of shoes or headphones, it's not selfish. It's a strong desire to fit in with their community. To bridge the protection and support that the parents are supposed to give, into a peer group "out in the wild."

One issue with these groups is that many teenagers seek a dopamine hit. Their baseline level of dopamine, which is the chemical in the brain that measures excitement, is low during adolescence. So, teenagers constantly find adventures and even danger to raise those dopamine levels. Lots of times they do this in a group.

Many teenagers find themselves in traumatic situations, not because they are craving drama. They're just looking for a hit of dopamine. What they, and their parents, don't realize is that it takes more excitement to release these "feel-good" chemicals at this age. But their brain also releases more dopamine with every opportunity.

It's a perfect chemical storm to create a risk-taking mind-set.

LET'S PRACTICE—LISTS

Dialectical behavior therapy (DBT) is a thinking therapy designed to help with borderline personality disorder (BPD).

I want to tread carefully here because there's overlap between BPD and complex trauma symptoms. But some people find the diagnosis validating, so it's contentious to claim it's always one or the other. Regardless, DBT is helpful for every single human on the planet. I wish we would teach these skills in schools.

One skill that is taught during DBT is called the *pros-and-cons list*. This is probably something you've heard of before. It's a traditional resource, to make a list of all the reasons an action is a good idea and all the reasons it's not a good idea. It's popular in DBT because you can generally discuss it in a group.

The twist in this exercise is to add a second DBT skill: that of considering what a friend might advise you to do. Looking at a situation from another person's perspective can be helpful, to get outside our own frame of mind.

Consider the last time that you were trying to make a big decision. One where there was a risk on one or both sides of the choices. Instead of imagining a pros-and-cons list that you would come up with, can you imagine one that somebody who cares about you—a friend, a parent, a partner, or a person you trust (at school or work or spiritual space)—might write. If no one would know you well enough, imagine an ideal best friend or parent. Or use a fictional character from a book or movie that's meaningful to you.

After you've done that list, could you think of another person's perspective to consider and write it out again? Did some new ideas come up?

Some of those thoughts on the list might feel annoying. Sometimes, when a person wants you to stay safe, it feels like they're wanting you to stay small.

The difference is, when you're framing a risk for another person, you see the situation more objectively. There's not as much emotion involved. What did you notice about their perspectives?

Brains

The brain doesn't finish its adolescent growth until about the age of twenty-five. Before that time, the frontal lobes aren't fully formed, which oversee *executive functions*. It means things like planning ahead, making rational decisions, and thinking about the future aren't as easy. This anatomical fact shows up as difficulty managing one's impulses or doing things without thinking them through.

And all of this is happening at a time when the brain is also forming its self-identity. Who you are, who you want to be, and what matters to you.

Here's an Example

José was invited to a party where he didn't know a lot of people. The friend he arrived with disappeared into the hot tub, so José kicked around the kitchen. He saw a guy that he found attractive across the room, who seemed to catch his eye.

The guy came over to him with two cans of beer, handing one to José. Knowing he was driving his friend home, he hadn't planned to drink that night. But he didn't want to seem like a loser to this stranger. And one drink wouldn't hurt.

The next two drinks went down automatically, without thinking about it. José chatted with this guy, who seemed interested. They go upstairs, and the guy offers him a line of coke before they hook up. José has never done coke before but wants to impress this guy and is enjoying himself. So, he tries it, and the next couple of hours are a blur.

He doesn't remember deciding to drive home.

It had always been the plan, so his friend hadn't thought to ask if he was safe to drive. These events cost José his friend's life and a lot more.

Potential

That was a sad, difficult story—so I don't want to end the chapter there.

The beauty of the adolescent mind is how fast it can be changed. Neural pathways are forming so fast, and the ability to learn new things is the highest it will be for a human's entire life. The potential here is amazing—even if there is trauma, there is the possibility to rewire the brain at the same time. Practices like empathy, gratitude, and forgiveness taught at this age help the brain form in ways that protect against trauma responses.

The last thing we want is for a person with an adolescent brain to feel helpless or hopeless. That, along with impulsivity, can lead them to consider self-harm. Truly, there's never a time in our lives where our brain has more potential. The possibility of growth is awesome at this stage of life, when in the right environment.

CHAPTER 9

Our Relations

Relational Trauma

There's a difference between trauma that happens from single events or even compounded events compared to the ones that develop from not getting our emotional needs met as children. Emotional traumas linger differently than shock and affect all our relationships.

When we're young, we need to get our physical and emotional needs met by others. And if we need soothing, generally a caregiver would soothe us or work with us to learn how to do that. If a child doesn't learn these skills, when something bad happens and the emotions are overwhelming, the child often dissociates.

This means that the child is no longer connected to the emotions because the sensations got too overpowering. This child that is stuck in this emotional state might become a part of the adult. In Internal Family Systems (IFS) therapy, they would call this an Exile—a child part showing up when the adult's past trauma is triggered. The emotions that were stuck at this stage reactivate and the "inner child" emerges.

All adult relationships have to deal with these child parts. Whether that's an ongoing connection with parents (if that's something you can allow), friendships, or a romantic or otherwise partnered relationship. These Exile parts of us can even show up at work.

Being in relationships with others, when you can't read another person's mind and their needs don't always make sense to us, is hard enough. Now, bring a traumatized six-year-old or twelve-year-old into the mix.

The good news is—reparenting is possible. And it happens in the context of all these relationships. Plus a therapist, if one is available.

Learning how to soothe yourself (if it's not something you learned as a child) is possible as an adult. And healing those child parts inside us that got stuck at the time of a trauma is, likewise, possible.

Feeling connected to another person—where you feel like they're trying to understand you and offer empathy—is a powerful experience.

Here's the problem—after trauma, though the person craves closeness, intimacy also scares them. If adult figures in your life have never been trustworthy or consistent, it feels scary to trust somebody and let your guard down.

Just like we create new neural pathways toward adverse events, we can also do that toward our feelings about connections. If all connections have felt uncertain and potentially unsafe, the brain doesn't want to get too close to someone. There's a sense of ambivalence—you want two things at the same time. You might want connection but also safety, while part of you might not believe that both could be possible, based on past experiences. (This is a core strategy mentioned in the Neuroaffective Relational Model [NARM]).

Yet, the more times that you can be with a person who offers you compassion and doesn't let you down, the better your brain can believe that this would be possible again in the future.

Here's an Example

Zahir grew up in a family where his parents couldn't pay very much attention to him. They immigrated when he was three, and while his parents had an education in their home country, neither of their professional qualifications were recognized, and they ended up having to work long hours just to make ends meet.

This left him to be raised mostly by his older sister as a babysitter. Being a teenager, she spent a lot of time on her phone and didn't really notice how he was doing. Zahir struggled with a stutter, and he didn't want to speak more than he needed to, in case it showed up. He learned to stay quiet because his parents were sleeping if they were home, his sister acted like he was a pest, and he didn't really bond with his cousins because his speech issue made him nervous around them.

Now that he's in an adult relationship, his default is to stay quiet. If he's feeling a powerful emotion, he retreats inside himself and doesn't share his feelings. It drives his girlfriend up the wall. She can tell that he's upset—he doesn't give her any eye contact, and he gets quieter than normal. But when she asks him how she can help, he just stares at the floor.

Zahir doesn't consider having a family—how would he handle kids when he can't handle his own emotions? He knows his girlfriend wants him to propose, but part of him just wants to break up and avoid the whole situation.

Attachment

It makes sense that when your primary caregivers as a child don't provide you with a safe place to talk about your feelings and a safe way to calm yourself down, the resulting coping strategies stretch on for the rest of your life until you learn a new way of being.

Some people say that the way to solve emotional regulation issues is through *co-regulation*. That's regulating alongside another person. I think that could be true, like with a partner or a therapist, but it's not necessarily the case for everyone.

Have you ever tried to look into someone else's eyes? What about for a long time, like a minute or more? The kinds of feelings that show up, from kindness and connection to terror and discomfort, can be surprising.

One reason that I was so excited to write this book is that I believe the healing of these relational wounds is innately possible within each of us. We can practice these connections.

LET'S PRACTICE—REPARENT

The next time you're finding yourself in a disagreement with somebody, let's approach the part of you that's feeling uncomfortable with some curiosity.

Let's not use a scenario where you're fighting with your parents or your partner, but something more minor—like a person at the grocery store, the club, or the dog park.

If you perceived this person as rude, maybe you feel an emotion about it? The first thing you would do is to notice the emotion. Is it anger? Is it frustration? What else could it be?

This doesn't have to be a conversation that you have with the other person; we can solve it by having a conversation with yourself.

We're going to imagine an age where you may have had a similar emotion. Maybe you were an angry teenager? Or a frustrated child? I remember being both things.

We're going to put that child in the chair across from you. What do they look like? What are they wearing? How is their hair styled?

This doesn't have to be said out loud, but in your mind, we're going to imagine that you are validating the way this kid is feeling. "I can see that you are feeling a strong emotion right now. That must be hard on you. I'd like to help."

Part of practicing self-compassion is to believe that it's available to you.

The next step is just holding space for that emotion alongside the child part. Let them know that it's totally okay to feel the way they do. That you are just going to be with them and be with the feeling until it passes.

"I'm so glad that you could find an emotion that signaled how you were feeling about what happened. It's good that you found ways to understand and experience the world. It can seem confusing, right?"

Let them say that it is. Because the entire range of human emotions is exactly what we should be experiencing.

Now offer them a choice. Feeling some control is important.

"What do you want to do about these feelings? We could kick a ball around. You could push against a pillow. We could scream into the sky."

Check out what this child wants to do. See if they relax afterward.

You might inquire, "Did you want to feel some love? I've got lots for you."

Imagine how amazing that would feel in this child's body. What might shift? Open?

Inquire if the child would feel comfortable accepting a hug. Listen to their boundaries and respect them if they aren't ready.

Always move at the speed of trust.

Service

New relationships can be hard when you've experienced traumatic ones. Mistrust, shame, and ambivalence might show up.

In terms of connections to other people, there are ways to do this that provide safety and also create happiness. For people who are wary of trusting somebody outright, acts of service like volunteering or helping could be one way to dip your toe into a relationship that has formal boundaries.

Research has linked being helpful to a better quality of life. It's often part of the journey of post-traumatic growth, to move from a mind-set where you wonder about your personal outcomes to being more curious about the collective. Moving from "What's in it for me?" to "What is being asked of me?"

This could be very simple and take place within your family (if they are people you're close to physically and otherwise). But it could also involve shoveling your busy neighbors' sidewalk. Or volunteering to drive cancer patients or newcomer moms to their appointments if they don't have somebody to help. The best way to do it is to combine it with something you're interested in and that you would enjoy doing.

What about taking tickets at a film festival? Bringing pet therapy to the children's ward of a hospital? What do you know that you can teach? What could you learn that you'd like to share?

Rejection

After experiencing trauma in a relationship, many people might face *rejection sensitivity*, so you're afraid people won't like you. People who experience powerful emotions or have different ways of being (like autism, ADHD, or high-sensitivity empath) might get rejected often, so it would make sense they'd worry about it.

Asking them to mingle with the public or make small talk might feel deeply uncomfortable.

With new friends or dates, such a person would be suspicious if things seem to go well. They might gather evidence of problems even if that's not the case.

It makes perfect sense from the perspective of a person who's been through trauma. Your attention is always biased toward the negative. You don't trust people. When we look for things that are said or done with this lens, it's easy to find. Misunderstandings mount up, which is hard for the other person. They might bail out, confirming the original belief—which leads to more expectation of rejection in the future.

The root cause of this is that somebody planted the seed in the mind that you aren't good enough. This often happens when you were a child, and every time rejection happens (or a perceived snub), it nourishes the belief.

We can shift all of these things. Through noticing times of connection, giving more attention and awareness to those instances, it will change our presumptions. Having a single person in our lives that we could trust—real or imaginary—is helpful.

Trauma Bonds

There's another common relationship pattern after trauma that can be noticed and shifted. The most consistent definition I've seen around a *trauma bond* involves volatility. It's pure chaos. It's high drama.

And it's not your fault.

We've already mentioned that when your system is overactivated, stuck in fight-or-flight mode, it may seek environments that are risky and dangerous to make sense of what's happening in the brain. This is true in activities that you do for fun like driving fast, even work environments like operating heavy machinery or choosing a high-pressure job, and it's also true in relationships.

The issue is that, if your childhood involved caregivers who weren't always consistent, and especially if they were frankly abusive, this might be what your child parts think love looks like. This makes the most sense if your gut instinct is already telling you that the person isn't treating you well.

As kids, we tend to assume that our caregivers will look out for us and meet our needs. If they are being unkind, neglectful, or even hurting us, there will be a part of us that might wonder why it might be happening. Maybe they're in pain. Maybe they had too much to drink. Maybe they had a hard day at work.

The most common assumption is that there's something we did to deserve it. Or that we simply aren't "good enough." This problematic assumption is where the emotion of shame comes from. And it's the underlying wound of most trauma.

When you read about trauma bonds, most of the time, an expert will describe that it happens in a relationship with somebody who has narcissistic traits. So, one person in the relationship is the controller, creating cycles of abuse and distance, then tries to win the other back.

A trauma bond is based on shame, where someone pokes a finger in the wound. Co-dependence, on the other hand, supports the behaviors related to shame (addiction, irresponsibility, or acting from the child parts). All of it stems from the relationships we have in early childhood.

Once we establish these patterns as an adult, it reinforces the neural pathways in the brain. People find themselves stuck in relationships that continue to traumatize. The cycle continues.

It really helps in the situation to make sure that you maintain your friendships. And make sure that your friends will be honest with you. Asking them if behaviors are normal, expected, and caring is the most likely way that you'll be able to see any relationship through a fresh pair of eyes. Alternatively, the friends might just be there for support if you don't feel ready to ask tough questions.

I believe that we often overlook our gut instincts once we've been through childhood trauma, because we get used to suppressing them. When we're stuck in environments that aren't safe, we learn to ignore any signals that we need to get out. We didn't have a choice at the time. Once we've started to ignore those instincts, it becomes much harder to rely on them as adults. You basically learn that nobody can be trusted, including yourself.

LET'S PRACTICE—THE CONTAINER

I'd like you to imagine the container where your shame belongs. Is it a box? A garbage can? Or a Tupperware container? Put your shame in the box and seal the lid as much as you'd like to. You could place the lid, but also add locks or duct tape or glue. Anything you need.

We're going to give this shame back to the person who gave it to you. Knowing that it probably wasn't theirs either, and they might need to give it back to their parents as well. One more reason to make the container really sturdy. It might have a lot of traveling to do.

I'd like you to imagine all the components of this container. How heavy it is, what color it might be, what's the texture if you were to hold it from the outside. You don't need to see what's inside it, just know that it's shame—and it's not yours.

Imagine a scenario where you would give this back. Do you leave it on the doorstep? Do you ring the doorbell and then walk away? That's my favorite move. You could also leave it in someone's backyard.

It might not feel right to give it to a person. Especially if you still have a confusing relationship with them, this might not feel comfortable. And I welcome you to listen to your gut on that. The more you learn to pay attention to your gut feelings, the more your instincts will send stronger signals that you can pay attention to.

In this scenario, you might want to send it on a rocket into space, drop it to the bottom of the ocean, or bury it somewhere. It will be up to you to decide where to bury it, how deep it needs to be, and how hidden this place is.

Part of this exercise is learning to trust your instincts about what you need. And part of it is imagining leaving this box of shame behind, knowing that it's not yours.

Hope

Although many of our trauma stories involve relationships with people who should have protected us, we can learn to be our own protectors.

The love and nurturing you sought from parents, caregivers, or partners is something that you can also offer. Self-compassion and an understanding of your self-protective reflexes are the starting points.

The next steps are noticing times when connection is possible and practicing new patterns. Just like any skill that we learn, trusting ourselves and then others needs practice.

CHAPTER 10

Loss

Shifts

The only constant is change.

As hard as it is to accept this, it's the absolute truth. And the only thing worse than getting older is not getting older.

When I turned forty, I visited the eye doctor, and she told me it was a matter of time before I'd need glasses. I had no problems with reading at that point and said that it wouldn't happen to me. She smiled knowingly. By age forty-three, I was in reading glasses for tiny print, with larger prescriptions every year since. Now, I have a pair of readers in every room of the house and in every purse. I can barely read anything without them.

Did I squint looking at the ingredients on a can of soup or lip balm for a year? Maybe more? Absolutely. It was hard for me to admit that my body was changing. *Degenerating.* What a horrible word.

Another situation that's been hard for me is the changes in friendship. People get married, then you don't see them as often. Once someone has kids, unless you have kids who are the same age, those friendships tend to wane. People move away, or their political views move further across the spectrum. People become obsessed with marathons or scrapbooking. They get busy. There are many reasons friendships shift. It tends to hurt more if you don't have a large support system.

With all the novel forms of travel, and the presence of social media, we are in an isolating time for humanity. Many of our ancestors would have lived in a single community; even within an urban setting, a lot of historical neighborhoods would have felt like a village.

Friends

There are times in our life with a natural opportunity to meet new people. Starting at a university out of town and living in the dormitory. Joining a new athletic club: a hockey team, hiking group, or Frisbee-golf meet-up. Taking up a hobby: singing in a choir, studying photography, or learning wheel skills at a pottery studio. Meeting parents freezing on the sidelines of the soccer pitch or at a student-run Pride parade. Having common interests is often the starting point for these relationships. But sometimes if they're built on a single foundation, they don't necessarily deepen. If a shared common interest is the only thing that you can talk about, it may not be the friendship that stands the test of time.

Research shows that your social network ties to longevity. Like if you were in a dire situation and the police or the hospital had to get in touch with somebody. Or how many people consider you a friend. Brief encounters, like chatting with the barista or a stranger at the dog park, counts as a social interaction that improves our lives.

Having somebody that you feel you could count on when things get rough is worth attempting to find. Is there a person in your life that you could call at two in the morning in an emergency? Someone who would post your bail? Someone who would take care of your cat if your apartment flooded?

Here's an Example

Maisie moved across the country to get away from her family. They were not exactly toxic, but she felt like she couldn't grow up if she stayed too close to them. Her *small self* always showed up whenever they were around. After the death of her grandmother, the person she had felt closest to, she decided it was time to leave.

She was interested in web design and took some classes online for basic website development. She launched her social media marketing and branding business before her savings ran out, but she always felt like she was living paycheck to paycheck. Maisie started working in the evenings to make sure that she had enough money to pay the bills.

She always went for a latte at a coffee shop on the corner, but some days, those were the only human interactions she had. At first, she didn't realize how lonely she was. She was too busy to pay attention. It wasn't until she had some regular customers, so had free weekends, that she realized there weren't many people she could call.

When Maisie decided she wanted to buy a ferret, she finally met people. It's an unusual pet to have, and there were only two places in town where you could buy them. She found an online community, and some people with siblings from the same litter would meet up. It blew Maisie away how her ferret, Jackal, always seemed to know her mood. He would snuggle across her neck whenever she felt sad.

Maisie's next project was learning how to play a banjo. She grew up in the South, and she winces when she hears folksy music now that she's living on the East Coast. But there's something about the way the banjo sounds that makes her feel nostalgic and wholesome. She chatted with somebody in line for coffee one morning who's a songwriter. They got together once a month at first, fooling around with the music. But soon, they had a standing gig every second Thursday on the small stage at the coffee shop. They even released a song on Spotify.

If a solid connection isn't something in your life right now, it's worth putting some effort toward finding a person (could you imagine asking any of your friends to be your emergency contact?). Think about the interests that you have, and a place where people might share those. After the pandemic, my suspicion is that a lot more people have made strong connections in online communities.

Relationships don't have to be defined in a specific way.

Some of the best ways to meet people are community teams or classes, volunteering, or clubs. There are online ways to find groups with similar interests like Meetups, or individual friends like Bumble BFF.

Sometimes social media means that our authentic lives aren't always out in the public. Sometimes people are comfortable sharing their journey with depression or loss. Sometimes, by looking at everybody else's seemingly perfect life, these truths stay buried.

Sociologist Brené Brown's TED Talk describing how vulnerability leads to happiness has millions of views; but it doesn't mean we're always comfortable in our vulnerability. Especially if being authentic about our emotions wasn't modeled by our parents or welcomed by others—it may not feel safe.

Grief

The human body supposedly peaks in terms of physical strength and functionality in our mid-twenties. But if a body is recovering from trauma, if their early life wasn't easy, the sense of power can improve instead.

Our bodies are constantly replicating themselves. Every cell turns over—for example, all your red blood cells renew within three months. Some organs are better at it than others; your liver can regenerate to an extent. However, the more turnover, the more chance your body makes a mistake. It was designed to handle those mistakes, to catch a cell that develops a cancer-causing error, but it can't catch all of them.

When the body changes, chronic illness becomes a possibility, and a life-limiting condition is the worst-case scenario—all these changes can cause grief.

In modern times, everybody seems to think most illnesses should be fixable and we should avoid death. So much of the trauma in medical training is the difficulty in accepting the limitations of a physician's abilities. We can't cure most diseases, and we certainly can't prevent death. But every time these things happen, medical culture makes physicians feel like we've failed. It's one reason I've seen people trying treatments for cancer that have less than a one-in-a-thousand chance of working. Or patients with dementia are placed on dialysis, despite having no quality of life left.

Cultivating acceptance and gratitude, no matter what shape your body is in, is difficult. But it's necessary to have a good life. And a good death.

The best book about death and dying that I've seen so far is *It's OK That You're Not OK* by Megan Devine. She was a therapist before she lost her partner in a horrible accident. Of all the brilliance in there, the biggest take-home message for me was to be very gentle on yourself with whatever it is you're experiencing. There is no normal; grief isn't a destination but a journey that's extremely bumpy, and best done if accompanied.

There's a notion that there are stages to grief after somebody dies: denial, anger, sadness, then betrayal, before finally getting to acceptance. Dr. Elisabeth Kübler-Ross, the physician who researched this phenomenon, was studying people who had chronic illness—not grief after a death. Her co-investigator, David Kessler, has since been speaking about a new stage that's vital to consider: that of meaning.

It's not that he suggested that there's meaning from the loss itself. But the meaning can come from having something in your life that was significant enough that's worth grieving. Or the meaning could derive from post-traumatic growth, how a person can learn key lessons about life and living from their pain.

Interconnectivity

There's a Buddhist concept of *Interbeing* that I cherish. The idea is that we are all (living and nonliving things) fundamentally connected to one another. In Buddhism, the pillars include a belief that suffering is a universal situation that we all experience.

Happiness is not the goal of our lives. Finding windows of joy and meaning is the only thing possible. We are all meant to experience the full range of emotions. That's the intended human journey.

Taking both concepts and meshing them, one of my favorite exercises is reminding people they are experiencing suffering—we can name it worry, fear, sadness, grief, or anything else. But it's only a part of the suffering that's going on around the world at a moment in time. Suffering has been part of the existence of all living things. It's something that unites us. We have part of the suffering that's going on—even when it seems like more than our fair share. I find there's something comforting about the idea that we're all connected through these shared feelings.

There are no negative emotions. That's all a perception in our mind. In fact, when they started research to find out what the core human emotions are, only happiness showed up on the positive side. If that's the case, wouldn't it be helpful to just think of each experience as more neutral? If we can change this perception, we can change how we experience it.

Let me explain it in more detail.

Instead of saying, "I am worried," I would say, "There is worry."

Instead of saying, "I am sad," I would say, "There is sadness."

You don't own any of these emotions. They are not your identity, and they are not the only emotion you're going to have in a lifetime, in a day, or in an hour.

Oddly, and likely for protection, the human brain is designed with a negativity bias, so we give more attention to things that are perceived as negative. This includes emotions. This includes things that happen to us, like when a person holds a grudge after one bad event, even if there were ten wonderful events before and after. It's part of our built-in threat detection, to notice if we're uncomfortable or in distress to try to prevent it in the future. So, it's not a phenomenon unique to trauma.

LET'S PRACTICE—LET IT FLOW

First, let's start by examining the emotions you have right now or the ones that you've had during the day so far. Sometimes, it's hard to name our emotions.

There are online tools and worksheets with huge lists for people to choose from. If you are uncertain, just search the words *list* and *emotions* online.

Now, we're going to imagine that this particular emotion is a color. It could be one shade of stones collected from a pebbly beach, or candies in a jar, or flowers in a vase. So, we're going to imagine that this container has many other colors in it too.

If you have a stone or some hard candy handy, you could do this for real.

(Although if it's a candy with color on it, you're probably going to have rainbow hands when you're done. It might just be better to imagine it.)

Picture yourself holding this colored item in your hand. Imagine the texture and the size and the weight. I love doing this with stones because there's something very grounding about holding onto something connected to the earth. Something with substance.

Whichever emotion you felt, this item represents the emotion. And we're just holding on to it for a little while before we put it back in the container and choose another one. While it's in our hands, simply acknowledge its existence.

There is...

I am noticing...

This is an experience of...

Multilayered Selves

There's a group of researchers in the Department of Education Science at the University of British Columbia. I met one of them, Professor Vanessa Andreotti, a few years ago, and we've become friends. She's one of the core researchers who work with communities in Brazil as a part of the Gesturing Towards Decolonial Futures (GTDF) collective.

One of my favorite ways of learning is through the body. When Vanessa was teaching us during a leadership course at the Banff Centre, she had us pair up and mirror each other in an enclosed space. Mirroring is acting as if you are in front of a mirror, so you would do the same thing that the person you're interacting with is doing. In fact, having similar gestures and facial expressions is a part of *co-regulation*, which is another safety cue. It's important for a person who's been through trauma to feel attunement from another person. Copying movements from someone perceived as safe would activate the *mirror neurons* centers in the brain. It's why many of us like dancing with someone. When these neurons activate, the mind feels "seen, heard, and validated." You might notice a therapist or teacher copying your gestures or tone of voice—this could be what they're trying to do.

When Vanessa explained the concept to us, and it's available on the GTDF website as well as in her book *Hospicing Modernity*, she described four ways of approaching our sense of connection. There's the mind that is self-centered and caught up in our own way of interpreting. That would be the ME approach. It can be selfish, one thing that makes a person choose their needs over another's or over the collective good. It comes from the teachings that we are separate—from one another, from the land, from all of nature. The singular ME reacts to the world from our needs and our experiences, creating the story of what we believe to be true and ideal.

Next, the ME AND YOU approach is to think of how we relate to another person, to consider their well-being and perceptions as important in the interaction. The same would go for our relationship with the earth, that we see ourselves as intrinsically connected. Not just for requiring the resources like food and extractive things to consume, but as directly connected to nature. The story still comes from the human point of view—humans own or enjoy or protect the land in this scenario. We still experience being *in a relationship* from a singular point of view. But we can hold common beliefs and experiences, create from a place of collective imagination, and live in community.

There are ways of perceiving the world that would be more Indigenous; theories that also tie to religions like Sufism or Kabbalah or Eastern faiths. The modern world has created a false separation between the human body and all that we interact with. It's like there's a grid of meaning with humans at the center, and we see our core self as being the most central. Technology and industry are the mechanisms that show up, and it creates a desire for growth and consumptive relationships. We try to get our needs met through the other living or nonliving entities.

The deeper way of perceiving is ME IN YOU, which recognizes that our physical body isn't limited to our skin. We're connected to the air, to the land, and to all living beings. Think of the trees that help make oxygen that we absorb through the sky. Think of the huge amounts of water in every body's composition, how it becomes recycled into the rivers and up into the clouds. It means that the pollutants in our environment sadly become components of every human, but it's also a joyful knowing of being a participant in the weaving of life. That anger, pain, shame, and well-being of this collective body affects everyone and everything.

The last concept is where things become formless. NEITHER ME NOR YOU is beyond time and space, beyond human consciousness. It's pure energy and possibility, the forces that create everything. For people who are spiritual, this is where the concept of an energy or force or Creator might play. Some people can access this way of knowing through altered states or holotropic breathwork. Some people believe this energy or universal consciousness is what we become when our physical body dies. We can only experience this layer of being when we drop our identity and intellect altogether.

To me, this relates deeply to trauma. Because it's something that happens not just to the individual but to the collective and exists within the universe. Even the big bang that created our solar systems has the energy of creation and destruction all wrapped into a singular event. These forces balance one another out.

For all the destructive and negative experiences in human lives, there are equally beautiful and inspiring ones. These are all times of possible connection and meaning.

Here's an Example

One of the most critical things that can happen from the perspective of someone who's been through trauma is the repair of a mistake.

Whenever someone feels unsafe, it's often that no one bothered to apologize or come to a place of understanding. Acknowledging and fixing a mistake can shift a foundational belief about how the world works.

In therapy, we call this *rift and repair*.

There are ways we can repair mistakes:

Notice when something has happened that shifts the energy. It might be obvious that the person is annoyed or angry, but it might be more subtle—they get quieter or have nervous energy.

Name the differences so that you are consciously aware of this shift. One could be curious about what happened, ask gently, or invite to speak about it. The other person may choose not to, so extend the invitation to another time.

Discuss the issue calmly, trying to keep an open mind and engage with curiosity. Remember that the "story you're telling yourself" about the issue differs from their story. To reach a resolution, the most important goal is to understand the other person's story.

Focus on shared values as the two stories emerge. What can we agree about? What parts of each story have common viewpoints, similar priorities, the same hopes?

Thank the person for taking the time to explain their perceptions. Sometimes clarification of each other's viewpoints is enough. At this stage, we might need to apologize—always choose this if you think it's suitable. Check in with your body to decide if that's available to you.

Unless there's a pattern within a relationship of always having to apologize for having a different point of view. That can feel like *gaslighting*, when your truth is always in question. In that case, I'd avoid apologizing and simply allow those differences to be out in the open.

Remind the person that you're always eager to learn more about their experiences and perceptions.

If you've apologized, stick to the promise that you've kept. Let them know how you plan to hold yourself accountable.

LET'S PRACTICE—YOUR CASTLE

If you're having to deal with someone who always upsets or angers you, it helps to form solid boundaries to feel safer.

In real life, these are the expectations you might set out in advance or the behaviors you won't accept from them.

To embody this idea, we can use your imagination.

If you were in a protective building, what material would feel safe? How high would the walls need to be? How thick?

Would you need a moat? A drawbridge? A guard?

Do you have weapons (cannons or arrows? I'd suggest not to use firearms, as that can be triggering).

What does your safe space in the building look like? Do you have a favorite spot to sit? Where does the sunlight land?

What colors are in the room? Do they change when you feel a sense of safety?

Grief and loss take many forms. Death and dying, illness and disease, but also changes. Moving to a new city, a friendship that shifts.

When we remember that trauma comes from the experience of an event, losing something or someone important can contribute to this response. It's when we look at the pain with an observing eye, waiting for it to pass (or at least change), that we can bear it.

And it's always easier to bear it together.

BAKED INTO
CULTURE

CHAPTER 11

Scary Times

It's a tough time to be growing up.

While most generations have faced war and famine, there are new complexities.

When I was a kid, we went through the Cold War. Everybody was afraid of Russia and the possibility of a nuclear attack. I remember watching a movie at school about the effects of a bomb. I didn't sleep soundly for months after that. It makes me sad that these fears might happen to children alive today.

Power

In modern society, people seek *power over* others, contrasted with *power with* (where you share). This is something I try to do as a family member, as a doctor, and as a person with certain privileges. With this book, I want to share some of the power that I have—knowledge and insight.

We've created hierarchical organizations where a leader makes decisions on behalf of the rest of us—both in politics and in business. Repeatedly, these leaders design situations that are not in our best interests.

I've been fortunate to explore other ways of working together. A *sociocracy* means people join "circles" of power that decide how to approach a problem together. *Holacracy* is a set of self-organizing networks within a company that encourages employees to be flexible in how they approach tasks, bringing their full selves to the table rather than an assigned role with defined skills. A *cooperative* is a group where everyone can join as a member to meet a common goal. These are models of partnership and shared agency, rather than domination and top-down control.

At the time of writing this, we are thigh-deep in the COVID-19 pandemic. New mutations of the virus are popping up every few months, which leaves many feeling fearful and hopeless. Simultaneously, climate disasters loom on every continent. Western Canada has faced flooding, fires, and other hazards. These weren't common when I grew up.

I don't intend to make it seem like everything is gloomy. A few of us enjoy the highest quality of life of any human. There is ongoing inequity, which results in many people still living in poverty. But even with poverty, it's different from one hundred years ago. Back then, when my Ukrainian ancestors first arrived on the prairies, they built a burrowed-out sod hut to live in.

Tech

My grandmother lived for over a century, so she saw the invention of the factory automobile and then the airplane and then the internet. It's hard to imagine how somebody could witness such significant changes. Does that mean we're going to be wearing personal jet packs to fly around in the next decade? I hope so, because that sounds really fun, but we can't dream of the technological innovations that will be possible in our lifetime.

Technology is a part of everyone's world now. In my travels, I've seen satellite dishes propped up on bamboo houses in Laos, cell phones tucked in Maasai tribesmen's cloth wrappings in Tanzania, and horsemen in rural Kyrgyzstan posting their tours of high-altitude lakes on Facebook.

Despite this incredible progress, it causes harm to humans who work in caves digging out raw materials for our computers or in fast-fashion factories with terrible conditions. It harms the non-human beings, most of whom are destined for agriculture and our food chain. This polarity affects all of us—the wonder at what we've achieved and the shame at the cost.

Exist

I feel like the collective trauma we hold is an existential dread. That means our existence has a sense of doom. It's like severe panic when we feel like our body is in danger. This dread is that "all things" are in danger.

They kind of are.

The climate emergency has created a whole new way of worrying. Similar to my generation who worried about nuclear attacks. The thought that our entire way of living might end, that all living things could suffer, is terrifying.

I wonder if the people making decisions that create these large climate problems are dissociated, which allows them to ignore the cause-and-effect aspects of the issue. In this context, dissociation is pretending something differs from reality.

Dissociation can also be daydreaming, distracting, and distancing. These are socially acceptable ways that we dissociate—not a diagnosis, but a way to cope. And that is absolutely okay. Let's meet where people are at. If that feels like the only safe way to be, to decide it's not happening or won't happen, maybe skip this section. I don't need to convince anyone of my opinions or force them into accepting something they're not ready for.

If being with the reality of the changing climate and what this could mean for the future is something that's ever on your mind, I'm in the same place. I think about it every day.

But I have a secret for you, something I've figured out through the mindfulness work that I've done. Not meditation—I find sitting quietly often brings out more worried thoughts into my mind.

We can hold two truths at the same time.

There is pain. And there is beauty.

In appreciating the small and simple parts of our day that hold awe, this is a healing practice. While things are changing, if there may be less comfort and certainty in the future, what can we notice that's of value in this moment?

Many practitioners agree that it's only in the present moment where we can be at peace—the past holds regret or sadness, and the future holds worry or fear. This is a brilliant concept when we try to deal with the existential problems we face.

What are the aspects of your daily life where you could experience wonder?

It could be...

The way that raspberries grow on a vine

The sounds of leaves rustling in the wind

A dandelion growing through the crack in the sidewalk

How a dog runs when it's missing a leg

How a face changes when it smiles

Snowflakes

Sunshine

Giggles

I love allowing myself to be held by the earth. That could be walking barefoot. It can be laying down in the soft sand and allowing it to form around your body. It can be leaning against a tree and running your fingers across the bark. We should think of the earth as all our mothers, as we are so intricately connected to her in our bodies made of carbon and water.

How does the earth hold you?

There is beauty and love and awe available to us. Even when things are hard. The more that we allow ourselves to pay attention to these small magical moments (Deb Dana calls them *glimmers*), the more we build the capacity to get through tough times.

Polyvagal Pandemic

The different reactions to the COVID-19 pandemic have been varied, and sometimes extreme. The polyvagal theory is a lens that can be helpful to analyze these.

When a person is afraid, the first thing that their body does is flip on the sympathetic nervous system to deliver a high-activation, fight-or-flight response. When a person shows up to a grocery store and screams about a shopper wearing a mask, this is their nervous system embodying this fight. This reaction can look aggressive, people yelling and calling others harsh names. It's hard to be on the receiving end of this fighting energy, as I was, because I did some advocacy work on the news. But I can find compassion in my heart when I think of it as a nervous system reflex, a response to danger. I might get upset in the moment, though, because I'm human too.

Once this high-energy nervous system has become overwhelmed, the low-activation state shuts everything down. This disconnect shows up as denying that there is a problem, despite facing solid evidence. As much as it's frustrating for me as a health-care provider, I can see why this denial is benefiting people to some extent. Dissociation is a valuable coping mechanism when reality is too uncomfortable. So, as much as I don't appreciate this line of thinking, because it has harmed so many people, I can find compassion in my heart for this too.

Another reason people might have these kinds of responses is a mistrust in scientists and physicians. I'll admit, we've done a tremendous amount of harm, while well intentioned. I've participated in conversations with families so desperate to keep a loved one alive that I agreed to set up tube-feeds directly into their stomach because I didn't have the heart to tell them it was hopeless. For much of my medical career, before I understood the power of the mind-body connection, I believed medications were the best solution to most illnesses. Now, I prefer to de-prescribe, whenever possible.

Medical training and becoming a doctor are inherently traumatic. Both to our body, ignoring signals for sleep or hunger, but also to our basic humanity. Maintaining professional boundaries is hard when sometimes we want to cry along with grieving children or give an opinion when a person seems unable to decide on their treatment options. I used to get so stressed out during busy night shifts; I was nauseated at two a.m. and my blood pressure was so high I could have had a stroke.

There have been many historical and recent examples of trauma caused by racism in health care. Some of the worst incidents include the time when researchers diagnosed syphilis in Black people but did not offer them the cure (penicillin), to follow the course of this horrendous disease (the Tuskegee study lasted from 1932 to 1972). Or the unwilling sterilization of Indigenous women when they deliver a baby (people report ongoing cases). Not to mention child protective services showing up at the least sign of poverty or substance use. These factors mean that, for many, the health system is not a safe place. Fear of harm from vaccines makes little sense for the general public, but it might, when you consider the historical harms within certain communities.

Listening to the stories shared with me by patients and on social media, those who are supposed to heal have caused harm. I'm no exception. When you've been through childhood trauma, this situation mimics being hurt by the ones who are supposed to be caregivers. There is bound to be more sensitivity. When a person is told their symptoms are not real (gaslighting) or not important (dismissal), that causes a mental wound. If someone has a disability or chronic illness but no suitable access into a building or a seating area, when they can't afford their medications or care accessories, or if there's a complicated process for income assistance—that's traumatic.

HERE'S AN EXAMPLE

Shanice heard about the COVID-19 pandemic through one of her neighbors, so she went on her Instagram feed to find out more. The first thing she read was that it was all a ploy to interrupt people's lives and make them follow orders that would harm them. She had been working in a call center; her boss told her she'd just have to make the calls from home. Luckily, they gave her a cell phone that she could use. She wouldn't have had enough minutes on her own phone plan.

Her three kids' lives were also disrupted quickly; two of their daycares closed, and teachers sent the third one home from school every few weeks because of outbreaks in the classroom. Shanice had to figure out a way to look after them while she was making phone calls. Sometimes she made the calls with one kid in the bath and another on the toilet.

Things got harder—the company cut her hours by a third because of a lack of customers. It's not like the landlord cut her rent by a third. Every time she checked Instagram, she read that doctors withheld effective medications. It reminded her of the time that her father showed up at the emergency room having a heart attack and the staff sent him home.

When the vaccine came out, everything she read suggested that it would be dangerous to put it in her body. The side effects, the claims that it wasn't approved, and the way it was developed and released so quickly made her feel uneasy. So, when her boss told her she had to be vaccinated once they were told to return to the building, she started having nightmares and panic attacks. She looked up online how to get a fake vaccine certification. Her heart raced anytime she looked at her calendar at the appointment, and though her employment was at risk, she tried not to think about it.

Many people also have a polyvagal "fight" or "disconnect" response around the climate crisis. It's the business executives who battle for their right to extract every ounce of resources. It's the industries that tear down natural forests and habitats who are in denial that the forest fires and flooding have anything to do with clear-cuts. Now that we are experiencing shortages of items like cars and cell phones, it's still hard for many of us to link it back to child labor in a mine on the other side of the world. Many of these mines are owned by North American and European companies, where the business practices they allow overseas are illegal in their home nations. This dissociation benefits shareholder profits, while it harms humans and other living beings. But this fight and denial is so entrenched at this point from these companies; with the blatant evidence of harm, their shady business practices continue.

Politics

Political polarities have always existed, but they seem to move further away from each other with each election. All sides seem to fight harder and stay in denial about the biggest concerns from the other.

One undeniable fact is worsening inequity. There was a time where we had a solid middle class in many countries, but that is disappearing along with a massive growth of billionaires. It makes little sense that so few people should own so much, but our systems have allowed this to happen. This is inequity that keeps many people worried about getting their basic needs met, putting them into heightened stress responses. This manifests as more people being irritable, using distractions like social media and gaming, and people comforting themselves with food. When these system-level problems seem beyond our control, there are small things that we do to cope and self-soothe.

Some of the greatest solutions have come from Black activists and writers. Octavia Butler, a science-fiction author who incorporated race issues into her work, made a beautiful comment during an interview: "There's no single answer that will solve all of our future problems. There's no magic bullet; instead there are thousands of answers, at least. You can be one of them if you choose to be."

adrienne maree brown, one of Butler's biggest fans, is a brilliant writer in her own right. My favorite book about systems thinking is her *Emergent Strategy*, which laces ideas about how to create change with poetry. One of her other books is about *pleasure activism*, how important it is to enjoy the work rather than allowing yourself to be caught up in the fight of it.

It's pleasant to come from a place of hope rather than a place of fear—you can dream and create easier. brown also hosts a brilliant podcast with her sister, titled *How to Survive the End of the World*—it's a lot funnier than you'd think!

Dr. Bayo Akomolafe asks, "What if the ways we respond to the crisis is part of the crisis?" He's a psychologist and poet who offers the course "We Will Dance with Mountains" that he describes as *postactivism*, to reconnect to our shifting world. "Where do you go when things fall apart, when home has been taken away from you, when the cracks appear?" he asks on last year's invitation. The class enrolls hundreds of people (he calls them fugitives creating local decolonial sanctuaries) around the world in each iteration, including an exploration of the ecopsychology of trauma, centered on Blackness.

LET'S PRACTICE—LETTER FROM THE FUTURE

Imagine reading a letter from somebody in the future. If you think you might have kids or if you have one already, you might imagine that this could be a grandchild or a generation beyond.

Decide what kinds of things this person might thank you for. Whether it's instilling certain values in their parents or ancestors, specific behaviors that you did, or major changes that you influenced.

We aren't all going to be historical figures that will make it into textbooks. Having that kind of expectation of ourselves just adds pressure and can cause our nervous system to get dysregulated from the weight of that burden. But we can do small things that trickle down into more dramatic effects.

What if this child simply thanks you for not giving up? It takes courage to bring a child into a world that seems dangerous and unpredictable. So many people have decided that having children isn't something they can bear, whether that's due to overpopulation or fears for their future.

There is no right or wrong decision around this, so perhaps this future child is thanking you for not having had children because a slowing down of overpopulation has allowed a greater balance between the earth's resources and what humans have been taking.

What if this child is thanking you for working on your individual trauma? Doing this kind of work makes a difference for future generations, whether or not they are your own children.

Even when the problems that we face seem insurmountable, there are healing things you can do within your family or your community. Healing trickles up through the ecosystem.

Can you plant some seeds of hope?

CHAPTER 12

The "Isms"

The longer I practice medicine, the more I feel like advocacy is equally important, if not more so, to the job. Many inequities and social harms contribute to trauma and to ill health.

It's discouraging to be caught in a disease-management system in medicine, rather than dealing with prevention or thriving. It was one factor why I studied social innovation and design thinking, which are methods to change complex systems.

To truly shift systems, the easiest entry point is to change the conversation. That's something we're doing together here. The next level down is changing policy and social systems that uphold harm in society. The deepest level of change is possible through internalized thought processes—the biases and assumptions we all hold.

These are potential leverage points where we can transform systems. More so, if there are large numbers of us working on them together.

The following exercise is based on the iceberg model of systems change. There's a diagram on page 270 with more detail.

LET'S PRACTICE—ADVOCATE

You've just discovered that your state representatives will vote on whether to continue coverage for contraception. You benefit from this support, as do many of your friends and family. But can your voice influence this decision?

The first point of influence is in the conversation. The government members are on Twitter, where political discourse happens. When you tweet about your thoughts on the benefits of accessible birth control, you tag your local representative and any other people who might be persuaded to change their mind. You might also tag any local celebrities or influencers to get involved in the dialogue.

The second point of influence is policy. How could family planning become an essential service? Is there evidence on how it affects the economy or social services? Does the government have a committee that deals with women's health? Do they have citizen action groups around family well-being? Is there an advisory council on contraception, and how are members selected? There are many ways to get involved. Sometimes, it means showing up at a town hall or council meeting. You might need to get on their agenda in advance or keep an eye on posting for committee membership.

The last leverage point available in this model is mind-set. How can you get more people to care? How can you help them appreciate how much this matters? The most effective way of doing this is storytelling. Many humans don't make decisions based on statistics and numbers, because it doesn't influence both their rational and emotional brain. But a story certainly can. You could make a short documentary about the effect of unexpected pregnancy on a person, their family, and the broader community. Show the impact on each person emotionally, physically, financially, and socially. Look at it from a *micro* lens (effects on an individual, such as an unwanted pregnancy) to the *macro* lens (effects on society, such as an increase in unplanned pregnancy rates affecting health services, family services, and the economy). Collaborate with people who will be disproportionately affected (such as students, trans or nonbinary individuals, immigrants, people of color, multigenerational families, and people who are unhoused, underemployed, or in low-paid work). Stories affect the brain in powerful ways and have a much better chance of changing someone's mind.

The world is unsafe for many people because of the "isms." You might be familiar with some of them—racism, sexism, classism, ageism. There's transphobia, fatphobia, and many other forms of discrimination. In modern times, there's finally dialogue about how these can create trauma for people. Separate from adverse childhood experiences, but often intertwined, they affect how we experience the world. (Ableism gets its own chapter, which comes next.)

An important related concept is that of *intersectionality*. Kimberlé Crenshaw coined the term when she described that belonging to more than one community of people who experience oppression would be additive.

There's a simple way to illustrate it. Think of the racism a young Black boy might encounter. What if he's living in poverty? What if he's gay? With every added concern, these are extra hurdles in a world that reinforces the dominant paradigm (what society considers "normal"). So, this boy would have to prove himself harder in school to be considered for college. He would be at risk simply walking down the street with a loved one.

Think of the "isms" as a steep hill, where each addition makes it steeper. This doesn't mean you can't succeed, but you'll need more effort and resources to climb. Some people might also carry a backpack full of "oppression" weight, so only extreme strength (and maybe some help) would get them up that hill. Other people have to run a mile to get to the hill, so they're starting late and are already exhausted.

I can see lots of changes already, in my lifetime, certainly much more than there were in my mother's lifetime and infinitely better than in my grandmother's. But we still have a long way to go.

Let's look at this boy closer. How many bricks is he carrying in his backpack? Where did he start walking?

HERE'S AN EXAMPLE

Dejon is in his last year of middle school. He wants to audition for the school play, but he knows this would put a target on his back with the other kids. He spends a lot of time at home watching gay kids do makeup tutorials and musical numbers on social media. One time, he stole his sister's makeup, to try one of those looks, but she got furious when she found out. She works as a cashier to buy those sorts of things because they don't have a lot of extra money. Luckily, she didn't tell their father about the incident.

Dejon plays on the soccer team, which he really enjoys. What's been hard to handle is the homophobic remarks in the locker room. The boys say things like "Don't bend over in the shower when Dejon's around." Sometimes, when they laugh, Dejon thinks they're talking about him, and he can feel his heart pounding in his head. He gets a headache for a day or two after a practice or a game. Sometimes, he has to miss school because the pain is so intense. His mom thinks he shouldn't play soccer anymore, but he doesn't want to give it up.

He would do anything to go to community college to pursue an artistic career, but there's a lot of family pressure to join his uncle's auto shop. He constantly worries about what his father will say if he ever finds out that his son is gay. Apart from a quick make-out session at a house party, he hasn't pursued any relationships. It's all online fantasy at this point.

Racism

Race, as a concept, doesn't make sense, but it defines reality for many people and has caused considerable trauma throughout history. It's well established through evolution that we're all descended from ancient ancestors originating in sub-Saharan Africa. Yet, there's a sense of separation from the people who journeyed north and lost the melanin in their skin tone. For every place humans migrated, their body adapted to the environment. Lightening of the eyes, hair, and skin was possible only because of the cold climate. Different stature and build were adaptive to different circumstances as well. There truly is no better body; we are all perfect adaptations to the environments where our ancestors settled.

The notion of race wasn't invented until it proved to be a political advantage. Once Europeans and Americans started kidnapping and enslaving Black people, they had a lot of incentive to ensure this violent and inhumane activity continued to profit. When white laborers from Europe were forced into the colonies, they naturally formed alliances with Black or Indigenous people. Those in power created an artificial differentiation where the white slaves would hold power (like a manager) over the Black ones. This was to prevent all of them from banding together to revolt. Sadly, it worked. The white people started to believe that they were superior. It didn't take long, one or two generations. The concept of race was established. People like my Ukrainian ancestors, who weren't considered the socially acceptable kind of Europeans when they arrived in the Americas (along with Italian, Polish, and others), accepted a social position alongside their oppressors in order to survive.

Although race is a social construct with no biological evidence, it causes substantial harm. Anybody reading this book might be familiar with the statistics of Black and Indigenous prison pipelines, victims of violence at the hands of the police, and the disadvantage of an unfamiliar name when you're looking for a job. All of these are established facts.

But what does this have to do with trauma? Many identify daily slights like mispronunciation of names or touching of kinky hair or "othering" as microaggressions. It's my opinion that this word isn't significant enough for the repercussions for people who experience these social violations. For some people, their body stays in the Window of Tolerance (ventral vagal calm), but for others, their nervous systems might send out strong danger signals—it's different for everyone and certainly not "micro" for some. A person experiencing this sense that they don't belong could believe that the world isn't safe for them. That's not "micro" at all.

The therapist who has done the most to date around how trauma is held in Black and white bodies is Resmaa Menakem. His Somatic Abolitionist movement and books have been tremendous resources for people to navigate these tough realities. I worry it would be appropriative of me to reproduce any of his work or concepts here, but I encourage you to check it out.

Being born into a *body of culture* (Resmaa's suggested way of phrasing "race") in a predominantly white country is dangerous. The life expectancy, the crime rates, the incarceration. Lack of access to food (something we call a *food desert*, when the easiest place to buy your groceries is a corner store full of chips and soda)—your immune system and autoimmune system are connected to nutrition.

So, what do we do about racism? Obviously, there are systems that need to change, and social innovation ideas could play a role by involving affected members to create new ways of interacting. One way is by using *design labs*—in Edmonton, a few hours north of where I live, they had a lab where they invited the community to combat racism.

But there are also significant ways that we can take action as individuals. If we are white identifying, the best resource I know is the workbook from Layla F. Saad, titled *Me and White Supremacy*. It's an unbelievably hard thing to get through if you're being honest with yourself, but deconstructing racism starts within each of us. Because these values and beliefs were passed down, racism is baked into our body and social systems.

It's so hard for me to accept, but if I don't, then I can't find it to change it.

Sexism

I don't subscribe to any of the binaries around masculine or feminine identity, so where I allude to the women in this section, this includes people who identify as a woman, female-identifying, or nonbinary. Those within the LGBTQIA2S+ community may face similar issues as well.

While women have gained rights over the last century, we still have a very long way to go. Sexual violence in the home and workplace is far too common. I will not advocate that we all learn martial arts to defend ourselves—in my mind, the key intervention point is how we raise modern children. The way we view gender has the potential to harm us all.

People who identify as men are told that emotional expression is not valued and should be suppressed. A more aggressive, less empathetic way of being is taught in a hidden curriculum. Humans who exhibit these tendencies rise to leadership positions, creating the belief that success comes from what's presumed to be a male characteristic. But it's simply not true.

Leading from the "softer" tendencies of compassion, nurturing, and support are powerful ways of modeling a different approach. Looking around the world, many political and organizational leaders guide from this dynamic with a lot of success. According to research, chimpanzee alpha males lead with compassion and generosity.

There have been some inroads reporting violence toward women. But all too often, the people who harm women don't get appropriate punishment and so the pain of the proceedings (which often blame the victim) can be hard to bear.

In medicine, women fill more than half of the training programs. But we don't fill the same number of leadership roles. The same is true in so many other sectors.

In my mind, the things that will make the biggest differences will be policy changes and shifting our beliefs. Ensuring that policies address sexual violence and intimate partner violence is worth pursuing, but ultimately, it needs to be prevented through cultural shifts in masculine norms. Political and corporate structures should value the contributions of women with equal pay and roles, but just as important is acknowledging that all humans deserve a chance to lead, so that we make these changes from the top. We need to serve justice to people who've been harmed—whether socially, emotionally, or physically.

Where have you noticed things that need to be shifted in your organization? In your community? In your family?

How can you influence the way that those around you, particularly children, think about gender?

Classism

I was debating whether I should call this section "elitism" instead, because it's the people who hold the most privilege in a society that are the most determined to maintain their elite status.

Many rich people believe in a *meritocracy*—that all it takes to succeed is hard work. There's an enormous problem with the bootstrap mentality, believing that anybody can achieve financial success if they're walking up a steep hill with a bag of bricks (compared to someone with no load on a flat surface). So many structures and a lot of bureaucracy create obstacles. A person who struggles with money spends so much of their day getting their basic needs met.

It's illogical to think that the burden should be on the individual to break the cycle of poverty. Society reinforces classism through nepotism and corruption. Also, it's easier to study when you don't have to work a night shift or to build a career when your family can buy your way into a good college.

Having listened to the experts, I think one step to dismantling classism is a *guaranteed income*—giving every person enough money to get their basic needs met. Many countries tried something similar to this early during the COVID-19 pandemic, with excellent results. It simply takes pressure off, making ends meet. With a guaranteed income, people can go back to school or pursue creative endeavors. With automation taking over factory and warehouse work, people designing self-driving vehicles, it's inevitable that humans won't need to be worker bees.

Throughout history, we valued different work. In the past, they revered artists the way modern times honor athletes. Scholars were celebrities. People fawned over poets; they were the historical influencers.

We don't reward modern artistic expression or child rearing or philosophical thought. If we want to improve our society, these would be considered important ways to spend time. Placing value on the work that upholds capitalism and hierarchies continues to harm everybody except the billionaires.

What solutions come to your mind? If you don't support a guaranteed income, how might we approach this problem in new ways?

Lessening inequity addresses many root causes of trauma.

Once the financial system stopped being linked to physical gold, it became "Monopoly money." Society agrees that a piece of paper or a number on a screen is equivalent to currency. But we built our systems on so much debt at this point that it's all become meaningless. If we need more money for social programs or an emergency, governments arrange it as debt or print more. If money has become so easily manipulated, there could come a time where the facade falls apart. It's happened in Turkey, Argentina, Zimbabwe, Iceland—and many other countries.

Monetary power structures uphold inequity. Rich companies and banks have a lot of political influence through donations and their network. Because of this, once somebody gets elected, they tend to uphold these power structures instead of dismantling them—no matter what side of the political spectrum they lie on.

Ageism

People who are very young or very old get discounted in our society. We only seem to value people in the so-called productive years of life. All of that's changing.

Despite the sad news we discussed about children's futures, there's abundant hope too. Kids are inventing products to clean the ocean. Kids are standing up for each other around bullying or transphobia and getting more equity into science education. Kids are inventors and innovators, and experts in the changing landscape that is childhood.

Elderly people retire and discover creative talents. Or they don't retire, staying in jobs while they find meaning and joy. They volunteer to create art exhibits or festivals. Older people are inventors and innovators, and experts in the changing landscape that is aging.

There was a time when human life expectancy was only in the forties. Kids grew up a lot faster and very few people reached old age. In many families, kids take on the role of parents when their own couldn't, generally because of a history of trauma. This carried the trauma into the new generation in more than just epigenetic ways. But these *parentified* kids are wise beyond their years. Imagine having to be a parent to your siblings or even your own parents. The skills around navigating the household, relationships, and raising your siblings—it means these kids miss their own childhood and grow up far too fast.

Education systems, job opportunities, leadership accessibility, and so many other systems do not allow these people at the extremes of age to have independence and decision-making power. This lack of agency means they don't always have the opportunity to contribute as much to the world as they otherwise would. Rather than a "Top 40 Under 40" contest, why not get rid of such contests that reward productivity and just celebrate the daily value that every person adds to society, no matter their age.

LET'S PRACTICE—THE MOVIE

This is a modified version of an Accelerated Resolution Therapy (ART) tool.

Imagine yourself at every age that you've ever been and ever will be. You could include your parents and past generations. Future generations too.

Let's invite each of them to bring a movie or video of a time that has been difficult for them to a place of healing. If it's an ancestor, this might be a black-and-white movie with no sound. People from my generation might have a VHS cassette tape recording. There will be movie reels, thumb drives, DVDs, and smart devices.

But you need not look at any of them. These younger versions of you get to keep their story to themselves.

Invite them to bring this movie, of a trauma that still hurts, to a big bonfire. If this doesn't seem right to you, you could also dig a huge pit or throw them into the mouth of a volcano. Either way, it has to be successful in getting rid of these images.

Imagine that a warm emotion replaces their pain. It could be love. It could be hope.

So, as we imagine these videos disappearing, it's going to be replaced by something peaceful. Butterflies. Sparkles. Flowers on tall vines. Just as post-traumatic stress rises from the ashes, these ashes are going to turn into something meaningful.

The butterfly has a lot of meaning for me. When I was experiencing some difficult changes in my life, a mentor explained to me how when a caterpillar forms its chrysalis, it's not a very comfortable experience. A caterpillar's skin dissolves; its entire body morphs until the butterfly emerges.

Post-traumatic growth was never meant to be comfortable. It's like you've walked through the fire, arisen from the volcano. More magical for having been through this transition.

There are inequities that create trauma and social positions that were given to us. I always refer to this as being *placed at risk*. Just because a person has been placed in a position of vulnerability, it doesn't define them or their capacity.

The people who learn to climb steep hills have tremendous strength.

CHAPTER 13

Differences

Humans were never supposed to be alike. The greatest benefit that we have, from an evolutionary biology perspective, is diversity. Different superficial features (like skin, hair, size), but more important, different ways of thinking and perceiving.

With modern medicine focused on disease, doctors consider any outlier compared to the average as pathology that needs to be treated. Sometimes, this makes sense. Your bowels move too fast or too slow. Your skin is too oily or too dry. But in other instances, it creates a disease where there doesn't need to be one.

When men invented Western medicine, the dominant person studied was an able-bodied white male. Women didn't get into research studies until recently (the excuse was because hormones fluctuate with monthly cycles). Black, Asian, and Indigenous people in America weren't adequately represented within the "normal range" of lab values (controversial race corrections are used in the US) or in the textbook appearance for skin conditions. In fact, what we deem normal in medicine is average for a tiny percentage of the world's population.

Let's examine the concept of body mass index (BMI) or weight-height ratio. A mathematician invented it over one hundred years ago to measure a group of white men. He did not intend BMI to be used as a marker of obesity; it was a metric for public health. Muscle weighs more than fat, so bodybuilders will have higher BMI but certainly aren't overweight. Someone could have an eating disorder but still have a normal BMI; meanwhile, they aren't getting adequate nutrition. Waist girth is a more accurate way of predicting whether weight might increase risk of heart disease or diabetes. But in medicine, we struggle to give up concepts once they're proven to be outdated—or even harmful.

This is one way the health-care system can be traumatic for people. We label a patient as different and assign a disease state when it's within a wider range of normal. We create labels when a person isn't functional in a capitalist society. I've worked with patients who are housebound but contribute to online recipe forums, the gaming community, and electronic music. One person makes cute greeting cards. Another looks after her grandchildren. Community organizing, urban farms, instrument lessons, or wildlife photography—there are many ways to contribute to a family or a society. One way is to value a person for being. The same as we would any other animal—not asking every dog to sniff out drugs or every horse to pull a cart.

It's sad that we only consider a person functional if they are traditionally employed. Simply existing is valuable. Working on your personal growth is valuable. Being a friend is valuable. We don't appreciate the work of parenting. There are so many other roles and ways of being in the world that we should recognize and validate.

HERE'S AN EXAMPLE

Sadie has been a wheelchair user since she was ten. She has both Ehlers-Danlos syndrome and postural tachycardia syndrome (POTS).

Ehlers-Danlos means her joints dislocate with very minimal movement. Not just her ankles or knees, even her hips and fingers. More recently, her jaw pulls out of place. When she falls, multiple joints end up sideways.

POTS means she falls down often. In this condition, her blood pressure is dangerously low when she changes positions, so if she sits or stands up too quickly, she might pass out.

It's a tricky combination. She's dislocated her knees so often that the braces won't keep them in place. Now that she's twenty-two, living on her own, Home Care puts her braces on in the morning and takes them off in the evening. Twice a week, they run an IV to make sure she stays hydrated.

With Ehlers-Danlos, she throws up often, but she hasn't figured out the pattern for that.

During the day, Sadie makes videos on TikTok about her daily routine. She provides hacks on using kitchen appliances with hypermobile joints. Or researches new theories and treatments for POTS, then posts updates. She tries things like diet interventions and online therapy programs, then rates them with reviews for her followers. When she's able, she updates her blog on her website, titled *It's Your Little Spoonie*. She lives in Philadelphia and sometimes gets recognized in public. One woman cried and said how much Sadie's posts mean to her and have improved her quality of life.

Spoon Theory

My patients taught me spoon theory. We should teach it in medical school.

Spoon theory resonates with many people who have chronic illness. If it's something you haven't heard of, it might be a helpful concept for you too.

The creator of spoon theory, Christine Miserandino, has lupus, which shows up differently in everybody who has it. For many, it's an invisible illness because you may not know a person has it by looking at them.

Christine was in a diner with a friend who'd been to some of her doctor's appointments. When this friend asked what it was like to have lupus, this confused Christine, because her friend had seen her crying in pain. So, she grabbed all the spoons off their table and some from the other tables. She told her friend that the difference between being sick and being healthy is having to make choices that other people don't have to consider.

If a person starts the day with less energy, it's like starting your day with eight spoons instead of twenty. Making yourself breakfast takes one spoon. A person who has lots of spoons doesn't need to think too much about what else to do that morning. Somebody with less energy and reserves will have to be thoughtful about what to do for the rest of the day. If you don't sleep well, that might take one or two spoons away. If showering takes a spoon, it might not be something you can do every day. Same with getting dressed.

Once these spoons have run out, it's not like you can miraculously find more. You might have to miss a meeting, so that you have enough energy to buy groceries or order takeout. If you cook, you might not have any spoons left to clean up.

Christine hoped this friend would understand that anytime she had to cancel a plan, or if she asks for her friend to come over instead of making her travel, it's to conserve spoons.

While she created this theory relating to chronic illness, I think it equally applies to complex trauma. If your brain spends energy avoiding or dealing with triggers, and if your body spends energy being tense, that's going to take up spoons. On days when you have to deal with sources of your trauma, like family members or ex-partners, you'll have fewer spoons to do other things.

I use this theory to help people understand they need to pace themselves during the day. If there's a symptom or an event that's taking up spoons, you'll have less of them to do other tasks. This is something you can plan for. If this metaphor is confusing, think of running low on a battery or gas tank fuel instead of spoons.

Recovery from trauma responses can create a larger reserve, which can help on challenging days.

Neurodivergence

This wasn't a word or a concept that I learned in medical school either. None of this chapter was in the curriculum back then. We need to change the structure of medical education to better understand patient perspectives.

Neurodivergent brains don't easily function in traditional education and vocational environments. This doesn't mean these people aren't smart, but the way we measure intelligence is narrow.

One way that society differentiates between neurotypical and neurodivergent is with the standard IQ test, which is deeply flawed. Now that we understand how a trauma response can divert energy from the thinking brain, imagine putting a stressed-out child in an exam situation. If this child has external pressure to do well from their parents, and internal pressure to do well as a people-pleasing response, sitting them down to take the test could fire up the amygdalas. Once that's happened, the thinking brain goes offline.

There are many other arguments against the IQ test—for example, it's not a predictor of future success. It also emphasizes concepts like mathematics and comprehension, while leaving out creativity and social skills. It includes material that might not be culturally relevant, like when a group of Australian Aboriginal children had top scores on a visual memory test but not the standard IQ test. These results make sense because visual memory is a key factor in survival when you live in a desert environment without a lot of landmarks. Intelligence isn't just cultural; it's situational, contextual, and time-based. None of this can be captured in a single number.

Now that we've blown the concept of neurotypical out of the water, let's turn to neurodivergent. Initially, this term encompassed people on the autism "spectrum," which implies labels on each end. When I was in medical school, these labels (like Asperger's syndrome) depended on the "functional" abilities of a person with autism. While we've scrapped these terms because of their ableist implications (and Hans Asperger's eugenics ideology), the idea of functionality remains embedded in the assessment of autism. Remember, to be deemed functional by medical professionals means participating in traditional schooling and paid employment.

The term *neurodivergent* now incorporates people who have a variety of mental health conditions that might make it more difficult to achieve success in traditional cognitive activities. Things like attention deficit disorder, dyslexia (reading difficulty), even mental health conditions like schizophrenia and dissociative disorders.

Anybody who self-identifies as neurodivergent has likely encountered trauma within traditional learning environments, workplaces, and within the health-care system.

Society has failed to appreciate the diversity of the human mind. So many people are diagnosed and stigmatized with these conditions that I think we forgot that it's advantageous to have diversity in a species. Neurodivergence also confers significant individual advantages.

One of the neurodivergent qualities that directly results from trauma is becoming a highly sensitive person (HSP), also known as an *empath* (not everyone identifies with both terms). This pathway forms in the brain when a child needs to "read the room" to stay safe. Training the brain to check for people's emotions and intentions can be protective.

Some children have to ignore their instincts about safety, as they're stuck in the situation. They learn to suppress their "gut instinct" and then have trouble knowing if a person can be trusted.

An HSP reads the emotions of everyone they encounter. While it can be challenging because of sensory overload, the skill can be a vast source of compassion and care. Many people with this characteristic are drawn to the helping professions, often becoming therapists. In this field, and indeed in life, HSP learn to ignore their own emotions while being highly alert to those of others. Some even become hypersensitive to their own emotions.

My suspicion is that attuning to others' emotions is one of humans' next evolutionary steps. Research shows animals like dogs, dolphins, and horses are capable of similar brain activity. It makes sense that it's possible for all humans, but we've suppressed the ability.

An interesting, related concept is that of *synesthesia*. Some people may see colors as numbers or hear letters as music. Their brain links two pathways that are separate in other people. I've actually met someone who had mirror-emotion synesthesia. They could read a person's emotional history and current state by looking at their facial expression. That's impressive ventral vagal attunement!

What if we reconstructed the disability model of neurodivergence? How can we make systems and policies, in schools and in activities to create purpose, work for everybody? If one-fifth of people are psychologically "different"—are these really "special needs" or simply "needs"?

Once it becomes apparent that evolution favors divergence, we will purposefully structure our community to welcome these ways of being and relating.

LET'S PRACTICE—SUPERPOWER

I learned aspects of this practice through Brené Brown's book *The Gifts of Imperfection*. The idea is that your perceived weaknesses are actually your superpowers magnified.

Let me explain how I understand it. I'll use myself as an example.

One of my weaknesses is that I can be quite critical—of myself and others. I have such high standards for myself, expecting impressive grades in school and making no errors at work. I hold those same standards to others—it's hard for me to accept mistakes (especially in the medical environment).

When I wondered how being critical could be an overactive superpower, I realized that I am conscientious. I pride myself on being thorough, making sure I do tasks rigorously and "cross all the T's."

It's easier to view myself with compassion when I think of this weakness (criticism) as an overactive form of perfectionism.

During the online course associated with Brené's book, I drew two versions of this superpower, showing that it's two sides of the same coin. The super version had eight arms juggling things. The more negative version was a witch with a pointed finger.

I'm easier on myself when I notice criticism—of colleagues, family, or friends. I strive to correct it, but I can see that the intention is to be conscientious and hope others are too.

How can you see your perceived weaknesses as a magnification of your strengths? How could you turn down the "volume dial" on this characteristic so that it works better for you?

A lot of these issues are trauma responses. For me, I was bullied a lot in school, and it made me want to be perfect so that I could get positive attention for being smart (although that backfired—being a geek intensified the bullying).

It's nice to identify these so-called weaknesses as ways that your brain is trying to keep you safe. If it's a part of the fight/flight/freeze spectrum, there's a clear link. But for something like perfectionism, that's less obvious. Perhaps I wanted an identity different from the bullies, so their hits to my self-esteem weren't so painful. My tactic didn't work completely, but it gave me a tremendous work ethic and good-enough grades to get into medicine.

How do these perceived weaknesses help you?

The point of this exercise is to foster self-compassion.

To believe that you are doing the best you can. I believe that you are. We all are.

Finding ways of being compassionate to yourself is an antidote to shame. Shame is the deepest wound from trauma. And often, it's shame that wasn't yours, but it lingers.

One teacher of self-compassion is Dr. Kristin Neff. She wrote a book on the topic and has posted some free exercises on her website. I establish self-compassion practices first with many of my patients. Much of this work is based on Eastern philosophy, which emphasizes compassion.

Once you realize that your brain is trying to protect you, that the reflex responses from trauma are adaptive, it's easier to understand that they aren't your fault.

CHAPTER 14

Chemicals

When I'm speaking about drugs, I will not ethically distinguish between the ones that I've prescribed and the ones that are currently deemed illegal. Any chemical substance can help your nervous system feel more balanced or throw the balance off. Illicit or otherwise. Drug use should not have a moral judgment, nor a legal one.

From my experience working at an adult addiction clinic, it's evident to me that most people who use substances (like drugs or alcohol) in excess often have a nervous system that isn't in a comfortable state. Either it's overactive, making their thoughts race and their body tense, or it's underactive, making them feel sluggish and stuck. I've prescribed drugs for anxiety and depression in each of these scenarios. But I also believe that people may take illegal drugs to ease the pain of these states—the pain of trauma.

Less than one hundred years ago, physicians prescribed cocaine and opioids. They would often take it themselves! The name "Coca-Cola" makes it clear what used to be in the bottle.

Locals encouraged me to chew coca leaves while hiking the Inca Trail in Peru. The guides claimed it helped with altitude sickness. In fact, many cultures have had significant knowledge of plant medicines for centuries, and it didn't become an immense problem in these communities. Opioids come from poppy seeds. One reason Britain colonized India was to gain control of poppy production. The countries where these plants are indigenous did not have a significant problem with them until modern times.

It's the modern traumas, of politics and colonialism, that changed the roles of plant medicine in our lives. The "war on drugs" in the Americas served racist and classist purposes.

So, when you look at the history of drugs, lumping the prescription forms with those that were used as traditional medicines, it's hard to determine that one form is good and one is inherently bad.

Prescription Medicine

Since I graduated from medical school in 1999, there's been an abundance of new psychotropic (brain-altering) medications on the market.

As I go through my thoughts on some of these here, remember not to change your own medications and to discuss everything with your prescribing physician.

I've seen countless people come off medications too quickly and fall ill. I've seen many others come off medications, assuming they weren't working, but then realize that they were.

When the DSM was rewritten, changes were formulated based on the available medications. Today, with new psychostimulants flooding the market, there's been much more attention on adult and child ADHD. While I know ADHD affects many people, I'm curious how much of it is caused by the speed of modern times, the additives in our food and chemicals in our environment, and how we expect excitable children to behave in a school setting.

In the context of trauma, especially complex trauma, signs of inattention could simply mean that the child is stressed about their home life or other dangerous situations. Poor memory and concentration make sense when your emotional brain has hijacked your thinking brain. Struggling to keep your emotions under control and feeling restless are signs of the overactive nervous system. Spacing out and being forgetful are signs of the underactive nervous system.

My inclination, when I see these signs, is to see if treatments for complex trauma will work before I add stimulants, which can mask nervous system responses. Although if ADHD is present independently, the stimulants might help the therapies to work. If a person can't concentrate, it's hard to get through a therapy session. There's no straightforward solution, and you have to consider every person as a unique individual—with no right answers.

Some medicines, even herbal preparations, can mimic symptoms of a mental health condition. Anything that speeds up your nervous system can make you appear anxious. Anything that makes you sluggish can make you appear depressed.

Caffeine, used to help people stay alert, can cause panic attacks in predisposed people. (Like me while I studied to get into medical school.) Energy drinks can also mimic the symptoms of anxiety in the body.

Benzodiazepines (e.g., Ativan, Valium, and Xanax) may be prescribed for short-term use in managing anxiety. My teachers described this class of drugs as having a similar effect on the body as alcohol. In fact, when somebody is in alcohol withdrawal, this is the medication we give them to curb the severe, and sometimes lethal, withdrawal symptoms. While it calms the body, it also can cause confusion and falls. It causes significant sedation in most people, so it would be dangerous to drive or be responsible for children. Basically, the same risks as drinking alcohol. Benzos are extremely addictive; I've managed patients who took them for fifty years and are unlikely to stop. Just as we wouldn't prescribe two or three drinks of alcohol per day for somebody who has anxiety, this medication doesn't make much more sense. If your problem is tension and a racing mind after a tragedy, it's a reasonable short-term solution, but it causes significant long-term problems and doesn't get at the root causes.

Another class of medication that is widely used, this time for depression or low activity symptoms, is the category *SSRIs*. This stands for "selective serotonin reuptake inhibitors," so they make serotonin last longer in the place where it's active in your brain. The chemical imbalance theory of depression states that people who are sluggish and sad don't have enough serotonin washing through the brain, so SSRIs will keep more of this chemical around. A review of studies in 2022 questioned whether this is the case—it could be SSRIs have another mechanism that may help, or it's possible that multiple pathways restore mood.

Most of the side effects to SSRIs only last for the first couple of weeks while it builds up slowly in your system, but it's sometimes hard to tolerate, because patients don't feel better at the time that they arise (some side effects show up before any mood benefit). A possible long-term side effect of SSRIs is the change to sexual function, the most common reason my patients discontinued them. For some, even adding a second drug (buproprion) doesn't prevent post-SSRI sexual dysfunction. We must use SSRIs with extreme caution in children or teenagers, because they can bring about suicidal thoughts. However, the risks may be outweighed by the benefits when a young person is stuck in a dangerous depression.

I find it fascinating that SSRIs are considered first-line for treatment of both anxiety and depression. From a nervous system perspective, one of these is represented by overactivity, while the other is underactivity. When I do therapy for each of these states, I use very different treatments.

Doctors might give people with sleep disturbance or delusions an *antipsychotic*. Often, this is a reasonable choice. But after trauma, sometimes these thoughts make sense as the body tries to grapple with stressful past events. The distressed brain might imagine hearing a voice to remind yourself that the world is dangerous. It might try to solve problems or reenact threats while you sleep.

Working at a refugee clinic and treating PTSD, I became more familiar with the use of Prazosin. It's prescribed specifically for people who have nightmares, to curb their frequency by dropping the blood pressure. Which is interesting, because another category of blood pressure medications (beta-blockers) can lower the symptoms of anxiety. How they both work in the body is by settling your sympathetic nervous system responses, the heart pounding and flushed skin. I've seen sporadic success with these for bad dreams—trauma processing is far more effective. It makes sense when you remember emotions are perceptions of what's happening in the body—if you curb the body's symptoms, it will shift the interpretations too.

You can see my enthusiasm for prescription medicines in curing trauma is scant. I won't speak to other mental illnesses, as that's not my direct area of study. Related to trauma, medications might mask the symptoms long enough to do therapy, but I haven't seen significant long-term benefits. There are theoretical paths where chronic brain changes might be possible. Imaging studies show that, for select patients, medications can remodel the brain areas that store trauma.

However, it is still important to note that they can cause significant side effects and many (some SSRIs and all benzodiazepines) are very hard to stop. They require a long taper (lowering the dose) to be done safely and to minimize new symptoms.

If you're on medications, don't stop or taper without speaking to your doctor. And if the medications are helping you—that's great news—and definitely worth continuing. If medications are not helping enough, or you've tried a few without benefit, know that it's a common issue among patients I've seen. This is part of why I wrote this book—to provide practical, accessible solutions beyond drugs.

Dreamy

I was a neurology nerd in my undergraduate years, and I'm still fascinated by the workings of our nervous system. Our brain generates enough electricity to power a small lightbulb!

Most dreams show up during the rapid eye movement (REM) stage of sleep. You'll probably notice this if you have a pet; their eyes roll back and move when they sleep. Humans are the same at the later stages of sleep, which is why you might remember your last dream if you have longer periods of sleep as REM lengthens through the night.

The best explanation I have heard about how dreams work is that, as our eyes move quickly, our brain tries to explain the reason they're moving.

So, it pulls from recent and past experiences, and makes up a story, no matter how nonsensical it might be. The action happens every time your eyes move; the dream shifts in that direction. People who've experienced trauma are more likely to have stressful dreams because those pathways are available and often explored.

LET'S PRACTICE—END OF A DREAM

There are people who interpret dreams, but it's not something I'm very familiar with. So, this exercise isn't about journaling for interpretation.

The key to this activity is the fact that you can't experience trauma while in a calm body. This includes trauma reenactment or flashbacks.

Take a recent bad dream that you can remember. Try not to have it linked to a significant trauma, because you don't want this exercise to destabilize you. It should be something almost surreal.

Try to remember any emotions that you woke up with as well.

Now, our goal is to change it significantly enough so that you change the emotion associated with the dream.

Think of it like this book. It's a choose-your-own-adventure. Because your brain was just making up a wild story, you have the option of changing the ending.

So, think about the parts of the dream that were not stressful, which could be the people involved or the setting. If both are stressful, think of a theme or color scheme.

Next, reimagine the dream as if only silly things happen. Give yourself awesome superpowers. Can you fly? Are you invisible? What kinds of secrets (gifts and weapons) are built into your skin suit?

Give yourself a potion to amp up these special powers. What color is it? Does it have a flavor? A smell? What's the texture as you swallow it?

Now, imagine a completely new part of the dream where it wasn't stressful at all. Change the middle, change the ending. But remember to make it as funny as you can. Some of my favorite ways to change this is to add monkeys or panda bears. To make everything animated as if it's a cartoon. Or turn it into a musical, with songbirds weaving in and out of the scene.

Check in with your body during this exercise to make sure that it's staying relaxed. If you notice that your heart speeds up (flooding) or you're feeling numb (freezing), that's your cue to stop.

Herbs

In studying holistic approaches to mental health through the Andrew Weil Center for Integrative Wellness, I learned about herbal preparations for mental health. I have limited professional experiences with herbs, so I don't feel comfortable prescribing them. Most of my knowledge about their success comes from patients who try them independently and let me know. These are some reflections I've heard, along with what I've learned through my course work. It's imperative to clear over-the-counter or herbal medications with your primary care team, as they can have interactions. You can overdose on anything, including vitamins.

Knowledge about herbal medicine exists because of non-Western cultures with long traditions of treating disease with natural remedies. Research into herbal medicine isn't in the interests of the Western pharmaceutical sector—which funds most medical studies.

There are many natural plants that may have benefits for helping anxiety: such as chamomile, lavender, lemon balm, passionflower, and *Rhodiola* (golden root).

Inositol, in the sugar family, has promising research emerging for anxiety, but the studies are small so far and the dose needed can cause stomach upset.

For depression, there is evidence around taking zinc and omega-3 fatty acids (fish oil supplements), vitamins B_6, B_{12}, or D, and iron if levels are low. The herbal preparations include *Rhodiola*, used by the Vikings in the eighteenth century to improve mood and fatigue. St. John's wort appears to be as effective as SSRIs (so are dangerous when taken together).

Patients tell me they find mood benefits from cannabis. Some practitioners have an incredible knowledge base about the potential use, but I've never been comfortable enough myself to prescribe. I know THC can cause insomnia and worsened anxiety, while CBD can improve these symptoms, so it's not true that any strain combination is going to be beneficial. Using it before the age of twenty-five can have significant long-term effects on brain function.

Herbal preparations lack regulations to ensure there aren't strange additives and that the active ingredients are present. This means that not only might the chemical you are paying for not actually be in the bottle, but undesirable ingredients might be present.

Trips

A major tool that's reemerging in the treatment of trauma is the use of psychedelic medicine. This sounds like a headline from the 1960s, but the racist "war on drugs" suppressed the research for decades. Despite studies showing that these medicines have far less impact on both people and communities than other legal drugs like nicotine or alcohol, these medications (like psilocybin ["magic mushrooms"] or ecstasy) have been kept under lock and key. The good news is they are being let out of the closet, with promising initial results.

I learned how to be a psychedelic journey guide with the intention of helping people through this experience safely. And while there are many clinics popping up like little forest mushrooms everywhere, I haven't started my journey as a guide yet. It's important to me that a decolonized framework guides the clinical use of these medicines, so we appreciate that Indigenous people have had a relationship with hallucinogenic plants for thousands of years.

This is probably why traveling to Central or South America to experience plant medicine has become very popular. Unfortunately, this opportunity has sprouted up a lot of nefarious people wanting to take advantage of trauma tourism. I wouldn't make any recommendations, because you never can be certain about the intentions and processes within a community. I will say safety is key and to get lots of references if it's something you're considering (and, of course, consult a doctor as these cause physical changes).

Likewise, trying to find psilocybin through mushroom foraging can be equally dangerous. Especially when so many mushrooms are lethal. Unless you're with somebody very experienced and willing to take responsibility for your health, I wouldn't recommend it. There are reputable companies selling measured formulations that are legal in some places throughout North America; soon, I expect governments to regulate these medicines.

Psychedelic medicine has been explored in palliative care (for a person who is anxious about dying). Psychedelics can treat different kinds of suffering. Enormous questions about what happens when we die and whether we have lived a meaningful life can be quite unbearable at the brink of death. Something I would call *existential pain*. A psychedelic journey can provide healing when a cure isn't available.

> What does it look like to heal when
> cure is not possible?

If you think about that phrase, linked to Dr. Rachel Naomi Remen, it can also be applied to complex trauma. You can't go back and change your past. It has already happened and created some foundational beliefs. But a complete disruption of your self-identity, a relationship with time and space, and a sense of interconnection with the pulse of the universe just might help. All of this is possible with psychedelics.

Again, remember that I am not being prescriptive because I don't know your story or medical history. But it might be worth looking into with a professional. Some people have very uncomfortable experiences. Others feel it bypasses true processing. Others are transformed.

I will disclose that I've had a personal relationship with this medicine, guided in a good way. I found it extraordinary how you can make a break-through in your relationship with your day-to-day world by journeying into a different dimension.

Some people have experienced so-called bad trips on these drugs (in the rave scene—ketamine is called Special K, MDMA is ecstasy or molly, and LSD is acid). That's because the most important thing about a successful journey is the set and setting. *Setting* means that you feel safe with the person with you or by yourself (your mind-set is the *set*), and in your environment. In my history with the medicines, I don't think I would have been able to make appropriate decisions or control my body during my journey. So, I don't think there's anything more crucial to consider than safety and setting factors if it's something you're wanting to explore. Context might even matter more than the choice of psychedelic.

Just Drugs

We've been getting further and further down the list of regulated medicines throughout this chapter. And I'm not going to call a substance like cocaine and heroin pure medicine in this decade (without acknowledging our com-plicated relationships with these drugs), though physicians of the past might have. But likewise, I want to honor that many cultures used these medici-nally in the form of coca leaves and poppies. There are Indigenous shamans who use plants to journey into alternate states.

Consider that, for most people who take something that is now considered a drug of abuse, they're often doing it in the context of wanting to shift their nervous system. Their drug of choice might try to make an overactive system calm down, which feels pleasant to a racing mind. If the drug enhances over-activity, that might help the numb brain make sense of what's going on.

It's important never to shame a person who is using substances; we simply can't know what's going on in their brain. While I don't believe that every single person using alcohol or drugs to change their brain chemistry and function believes they have experienced trauma, I know they have all experienced stress. When it comes to intergenerational trauma, sometimes it's a feeling that they can't express, but it lives in their head.

Not everyone who takes these substances finds themselves in addictive patterns—which suggests a compulsion to use, even when it's affecting their life in negative ways. But some people will find themselves craving, seeking, and damaging their relationships because of a powerful desire for the drug. Others will have a simple, pleasant experience. Dr. Carl Hart is a researcher who argues that people can use many drugs as a hobby without becoming addicted.

HERE'S AN EXAMPLE

Many of us have cravings and compulsions.

I have a sweet tooth. While I tell myself not to buy sugary treats, they somehow find their way into my pantry and freezer.

When I have a rough day, eating ice cream or pastry is something I do to self-soothe. The chemicals released from eating sugar will do that.

What cravings do you face?

In what way do they affect your life? Think of relationships, work, school, finances, legal issues, sleep, and time spent on it.

In what way do they serve you? What is working for you when you think about this craving?

What other ways could you solve this same problem?

Harm Reduction

The most important first step in treatment is compassion and self-compassion. Next is something that we in medical practice call *harm reduction*. Meeting a person where they're at, whether it's using a substance daily or trying to cut back. Finding ways to be less harmful to the brain and body while still feeling safe. For some people, what goes on in their brain is worse than taking a substance to turn off those dangerous patterns.

The story we're told by governments and most policy-makers, outside of Portugal, is that the illicit drug industry is harmful. And it is—the opioid epidemic has shattered lives all over the world because it's becoming more and more lethal.

Part of the policy advocacy that I do is to help push for the harm reduction model that provides a safe supply in a safe place for people who have found drugs as a solution—whether it's a replacement or a pharmaceutical version of what they take. There are companies around that will check the chemical composition in a sample of drugs, to make sure they aren't laced with more dangerous ones—that's harm reduction too. Drugs are a solution for people when they haven't found a better solution yet.

My work in addiction treatment involves helping people find these safer solutions.

And my advocacy work on social media and news interviews includes trying to help take the stigma away from this choice. Trying to convince decision-makers that possession of drugs for personal use should not be a criminal act. Especially when these "crimes" send people who are Black, Indigenous, or otherwise racialized to prison—while the people taking cocaine in bathroom stalls of major corporations face no punishment at all.

Frankly, the pharmaceutical industry is partially responsible for the opioid crisis. Physicians are also responsible. In medical school, we were told not to ignore pain as the "fifth vital sign" to assess health, along with heart rate and temperature. They encouraged us to use narcotics generously to manage pain—I remember being taught that it was a different pathway involved when pain was present and that they could not become addictive. During my early practice, I remember these words leaving my mouth, convincing patients who were nervous to start. It makes me shudder now to think about it.

Likewise, I think we need to be cautious with the medical management of trauma. Fortunately, there aren't a lot of drug companies saying that they can successfully treat PTSD with their medications. But if a trial comes to pass, including those from psychedelics, just remember companies poised to sell the medications fund most clinical trials. They don't have to publish negative findings, so any trials that aren't successful just get tossed in a drawer never to be seen by the public. So, it's important to be both open-minded and cynical when you're exploring what might be of benefit.

The best indicator of what's working is to become an expert in your own nervous system. That way, you can tell if you are safely navigating away from the overactivated and underactivated states of a danger response. If something is helping you, you'll spend more and more time in your calm and restful, safe-feeling nervous system, regardless of whether this medication comes in a tablet with a stamp on it.

CHAPTER 15

Media

We live during an age of incredible explosions of information and technology. In my lifetime, I saw the invention of the internet and then smartphones. My grandmother, during her 104 years, gave me her pedal-driven sewing machine. It's hard to imagine what could be next, but it's awe-inspiring.

I remember graduating from university and heading to Europe for a couple of months, using a torn, stained Lonely Planet book to navigate between hostels. The only way I could contact home was to get a local calling card and find a phone booth. Travel sure has changed.

Reality Bites

These days, we can hear the screams of people escaping a military crackdown in their city on the news. We see police brutality in real time. We watch on social media as natural disasters occur, people fleeing in terror, anywhere in the world. Although this capability has allowed us to see beauty and wonder everywhere, we also see horror and mayhem.

The brain is more prone to notice negative events, which is our bias—looking out for danger and problems to avoid them in the future. So, it's a safety mechanism. But it's also uncomfortable, because it means the negative stuff you watch gets absorbed to a greater extent than the positive. For every five news articles that you see about good things, your brain is more likely to remember the one that's scary. Let's not even get into a discussion about who owns most news stations and newspapers. Or how

155

Facebook manipulates our newsfeed, or the FYP (for you page) on TikTok bans accounts run by activists more than it does racists.

All this negativity can feel overwhelming. Learning about the climate or financial crisis and other awful events can push our nervous systems into either the overactive or the underactive mode.

Some of my friends take breaks from the news. That's one solution. But it means they aren't as informed when policies change, or transformational things happen in the world. Likewise, some people only pay attention to what's happening locally. But there's inspiring news around the world.

Global Digest

TikTok has creators from every country; sometimes I'm surprised when a person has been modeling clothes or dancing—then I find out they live on the other side of the planet, and I marvel at our connection. One of my favorite pages on Facebook is called "View from My Window." People post their views and a short story about their lives. It gives me a sense of interconnection. Last year, Ukrainians posted their views right before the invasion by Russia, and thousands of people offered words of comfort.

I've lived for many months in countries like Laos and Nepal. This gives me the fortunate firsthand experience of knowing that our way of living in the Americas and Europe is unique. While we have more access to things to buy, many of us have less access to a genuine community.

ABCD

I spent a week learning from John McKnight in Montreal about his concept of asset-based community development (ABCD) and the local solutions. What this means is, instead of looking at a community to fix its pressure points and vulnerabilities, you look for its strengths and resources.

It's easy to use the lens of the traumas a community has faced. Especially when those are systemic, like poverty and crime. When you look at the roots of these, there is often deep ancestral trauma and ongoing discrimination. How can we look at this from a positive perspective? Working with refugees, I've witnessed the closeness of their family ties and how many connect to their ancient practices. They might have a culture that celebrates using music or dance. They might cook together in small kitchens while their kids run underfoot. They might have weddings and celebrations so big that it seems they have invited an entire village.

Just as many of the traumatic events we face are collective, healing can happen altogether in the same way. Taking an ABCD approach helps us learn from one another. And social media is one of those places where learning can happen.

Medium

Sometimes, the media feed contributes to pain. Seeing all the airbrushed bodies on Instagram can be distressing to a person who doesn't eat in healthy patterns. While the brain tells you it's not real, it's hard to deny what your eyes are seeing. The aspirational posts of a person "living their best life"—whether that's traveling to sunny beaches or having a picture-perfect family—don't show you the challenges they're facing. It just makes you feel bad when you're struggling.

Seeing violence can desensitize us to it. Either gaming or news media can present it as a normal phenomenon. Especially when we see it perpetrated on a particular community, this compounds biases and racism.

Other types of posts, about mental health and trauma, can be influential in multiple ways. On the one hand, I've seen lots of people self-diagnose with autism, ADHD, or PTSD based on symptoms described online—someone has coined the term "cyberchondriac." While I don't think the DSM exactly hits all the marks, this overdiagnosis concerns me because these people could end up on a medication for life that isn't necessary. Especially if there can be other tools that are useful if the problem is actually an overactive or underactive nervous system. On the other hand, many people wouldn't have access to a diagnosis without hearing about the symptoms they share through social media. Especially in the case of women or people from different cultural backgrounds, when their presentation may not be flagged by a primary care team. The first time they might feel understood and validated could be a social media post.

Yet, consider the privilege of having access to a professional for diagnosis—these resources aren't available to all people, so their only option is to figure it out alone. I also acknowledge that many people with lived experience do excellent research and often know more than the professionals about their own condition—we need to be more curious and humble in health care.

When we consider the concept of ABCD, one of the beautiful things that social media can do is create a community. A community of practice, learning, and support. The availability of information is so staggering that it can feel like you're drinking from a fire hose. But if you can stagger the times instead of binge, and be deliberate about what you are exploring, it can be helpful. Even healing.

LET'S PRACTICE—CHECKING IN

Decide if your social media exploration is doom-scrolling or hope-finding by listening to your nervous system.

No matter which social media platform you use, how does your body feel while you're on it? How does it feel once you log off?

This is one reason I switched my main scrolling to TikTok, because I felt like their algorithm helped me curate my page. If I'm having a stressful day, one of my favorite things to do is to watch a live musician or pottery on TikTok. There are also a lot of channels that are focused on relaxation methods.

How does your body feel while you are watching dancing? A makeup tutorial? Children or pets doing silly things?

When your body is overactive and restless, what brings it into a better balance?

When your body is underactive and flat, what activates you?

Then, how do you pull yourself away? When your nervous system feels overloaded, it can be easy to spend hours on social media blocking out reality.

I've set a timer on my devices and on the app itself to let me know how much time has passed. So, I have to really deliberately ignore it if I'm going to go beyond a certain number of minutes. If I'm mindlessly scrolling, it serves as a bit of a wake-up call.

Celebrity

The book by leadership expert Meg Wheatley, *Who Do We Choose to Be?*, impacted me because she tells the straight truth about the dilemmas we face. In it, she describes the sadness of feeling that our way of life is changing. She calls it the downfall of a civilization. She noted one marker when societies crumble, that of celebrity.

While it's ridiculous that people can inherit billions of dollars, or make billions selling expensive medications or online junk, it makes no sense that we pay millions of dollars to a pop singer or athlete. Their work in the world is of value and significance, brings joy to lots of people, and showcases their talents. But I struggle to see how it's a more important role than that of a teacher or a nurse.

Meg describes the focus on celebrity as something that allows an entire culture to become distracted. When we're glued to our television watching our sports team, following our favorite movie stars on their social media feed, or listening to our favorite album on repeat—it's an easy way to dissociate. It's also socially acceptable; nobody is going to fault you for spending time watching a reality TV show because they're probably doing the same thing.

Celebrity culture can be a point of pride—such as in the LGBTQIA2S+ community that values icons who represent authenticity and bravery. Likewise, watching sports can build camaraderie, helping people co-regulate and bond as they cheer their favorite players. It all depends on how we engage with celebrities, whether it's helpful or harmful.

The problem is excess. If a person is spending so much time gaming that they lose track of the last time they showered, that's not ideal. Or if somebody is so convinced that they can be a star athlete or famous singer that they drop out of school—but then don't have a realistic plan to work toward their goal.

Here's an Example

Jun has dreams about accolades from her fans. As soon as she wakes up, she checks her Instagram feed for interactions and growth. Then, she thinks about the content she wants to create that day.

She has a job working as an accountant for an electric company. But it's so boring! Any spare minute she has—she's checking Instagram.

Sometimes the posts get on her nerves. Jun lives in a wheelchair and gets bothered by all the ableism she sees online. There's also a lot of appropriation of her traditional heritage, which is both Filipina and Native American. Anytime she sees a person adopting something from her culture without knowing the significance and explaining its origin, there's an explosion in her brain.

It feels like a teakettle that's whistling out her ears. Sometimes she writes in all caps about how awful the creator is and explains where the tradition comes from. When she's furious, she misspells words because her thinking brain isn't working. She's gotten banned twice, which really messes with the algorithm and her growth on the app.

She tried a digital detox last year, but it didn't go very well. She still thought about her socials all the time, wondering what her favorite pages were featuring, but mostly feeling lost and empty.

What Is Normal, Anyway?

One fascinating psychotherapy concept around dissociation is the idea of a difference between our personalities that are the apparently normal part (ANP) and the emotional part (EP). It's most socially acceptable to interact with each other and on social media as an "apparently normal" person. But more and more, there's allowing for authenticity and being exactly who we are.

When the EP is being genuine, it helps others relate. Because humans experience every single emotion. And if someone's EP focuses their content on solutions they discovered, that's helpful for everybody reading or watching.

The kicker is when social media favors the ANP. It leads people to airbrush and fake happiness, as if it's the only emotion they feel. When you're showing up with fraudulent bravado and pretend smile in the world, that can be exhausting. People have exposed content creators for faking their story; one woman in Australia pretended to recover from cancer to sell theories about healthy eating. Others have broken down from the pressure of pretending to be in a good mood all the time.

"Good vibes only" is a common phrase. And it makes sense, because when we're feeling fragile or wounded, it's hard to have a mean-spirited conversation around you. But it can also lead to *toxic positivity*, where the full range of human emotions isn't welcome.

LET'S PRACTICE—BEING SOCIAL

How do you keep your social media feed free of trolls while still showing what matters to you?

One way is to showcase your beliefs in your bio.

Are you liberal or conservative? How important is the Black Lives Matter movement to you? Do you want to acknowledge that you live on the traditional territory of Indigenous people? A couple of well-placed emojis can create a vibe.

When somebody is harassing you, can you distance yourself from the comments and not take it personally? Think of the state their own nervous system must be in, likely overactivated and angry, in order to make such a statement. They're trying to create the same reaction in you in order to dissipate their own energy. You might decide to rise to that level of agitation, but chances are that it will keep coming back and become an exhausting interaction.

Would it help if a pinned comment includes a boundary around an acceptable way to discuss your content? You might want to say "good vibes only," if that's best for you.

Another option is to write:

"I welcome learning about your perspectives and I'm curious about your thoughts."

"Personal attacks on me or my contacts are not welcome and will be deleted."

"I'm creating a *safe space* for everybody who visits my page."

Remove the Masks

The capitalist lifestyle model produces comfort as well as great harm. Passing through traditional education systems and then joining the hamster wheel of productive work is the path for most people. We all have to pay tax and get our basic needs met in the system.

Sadly, the modern financial system leaves out people who are neurodivergent. Social media is a place where they can find community, acceptance, and even earn money.

Neurodivergent people face pressure to mask their symptoms, or pretend that they don't have them, to get by in the world. This can take a lot of spoons. And then it leads to the confusion of having your EP personality available when you're alone or with close people in your life, and a completely different ANP persona in public.

Wouldn't it be incredible if everybody felt safe to just be themselves?

If you were in a meeting in an accepting boardroom, picture one person spinning in their chair, *stimming* (self-stimulating through movement or noise, common with autism). Another might use a bubble popper to calm their anxiety. And a third wears headphones so that people's voices aren't so loud.

Your entire self, all of your quirks and needs, is welcome here.

SOMATICS

CHAPTER 16

Senses

These next five chapters focus on somatic, or body-based, processes.

As mentioned, there are two pathways into modifying trauma reflexes: *top-down* cognitive paths use your brain to influence the mind-body system. *Bottom-up* somatic paths use your body to shift the mind-body system— something easy and low-risk to learn. This is what we'll explore here, starting with the senses.

Pay attention to avoid flooding or freezing, in case the practices are dysregulating. Then, take something else off the menu here. Remember— the key is relearning how to be in a calm body. One of my teachers, Dr. Eric Gentry, says that you can't reexperience trauma responses in a calm body.

Attune

One of the important facets of the polyvagal theory has to do with the vagus nerve—cranial nerve ten (X), which signals to and from the face. Its job includes telling your brain information about how parts of your head and neck are feeling, from your ear canal to your throat. It provides some of the motor signals to tell you to move your voice box (larynx), as well as the upper parts of your throat that help swallow.

Because this nerve relates to our voice, it means that a person checking if another human or animal is safe will pay attention to their voice. High pitched and shrill can signal that a person is in danger, whereas low pitched and raspy creates signs of danger in the listener.

Vocal prosody (the singsong quality of one's voice) is a key component to deciding if another person is safe or not. It's why using a melodic (up and down movements) soft voice would be typical with a baby or a pet. This processing is part of the calm ventral vagal system—looking for facial expressions and tone of voice to determine if the person you're speaking with is safe.

Unfortunately, when a child grows up in a situation that wasn't consistently attuned, they can't "fight or flight" away. They might mistrust or ignore the instincts telling them when they could be in danger. Learning to trust one's "gut" again is part of trauma therapy.

Alternatively, a child with an inconsistent home might become careful and aware. Being *hypervigilant* is one of the criteria to define PTSD—looking over one's shoulder and being jumpy. But when someone can harness the power of this vigilance, they can tune in to another person's energy without getting overwhelmed. This is "reading the room"—one trait of an empath.

Here's an Example

When Rory was three, her father lost his job. Being in sales was his identity, and he was distraught. He always had a drink or two to celebrate a big day of commissions. But he wasn't celebrating anymore. He started drinking when he woke up. All Rory knew was that her fun dad was gone.

When she tried to get him to play with her, he'd bat her hand away. A couple of times, he growled at her. She listened to him yelling at her mom late at night. Sometimes, Rory imagined she floated away on a pink unicorn cloud. Her dad's voice sometimes shattered through the cloud and she crashed back into her room. She hid, shivering, under the bedcovers.

Now that Rory is a teenager, anytime she hears a raised or growling voice, it brings her right back to those feelings. Fear, worry, and betrayal. Although her parents separated years ago, and her dad remarried and has a new job, there's a part of her that still feels like a little girl hiding in her room.

When this happens, Rory shuts down. Her eyes go blank and she doesn't speak. She tries to leave the situation as fast as she can. Once, when her best friend yelled at her, she snuck a couple of cans of beer from her dad's TV fridge in his basement. He was so busy with his new family that he didn't notice.

Rhythm

Just as the voice can be a source of danger, many sounds can be a source of peace. It really depends on the person. I find Celtic music soothing; it reminds me of records that my dad used to play. Bagpipes—not so much.

Others find crystal or metal bowls very calming—a deep hum comes from those when you run a felt (or wood) mallet across the rim. This is sometimes called a *sound bath*, a total immersion of the body with this resonance. Every cell responds to the sound that you're hearing, not just the ear that signals your brain. You feel the vibrations in your bones.

Drumming is also a powerful sensation, both to be in rhythm with other people in a drum circle and to be inside the circle and feeling the sound reverberate off your entire being. Rhythmic movement, specifically when it involves both sides of your body, creates a channel between each half of your brain. This is because the left half of your brain oversees the movements of the right side of your body (except the face) and vice versa. The prominent psychiatrist and trauma expert Dr. Bruce Perry says that rhythm is a critical path to healing.

Bilateral stimulation, movement on both sides, helps our brain become calm. When you listen with earphones, it can be delightful when each side plays something different. People create 8D/16D music (which sounds like it moves in a circle all around you) by slowly panning the stereo field from one side to the next. This is different from 3D music, which has separate tracks in each ear. Many people with autism or other neurodivergence find the extra dimensions pleasing.

These *binaural beats*, where the audio alternates between the left and the right, can create a calming effect. They're easy to search for on YouTube; they label some specifically for anxiety or for insomnia. I would hesitate to recommend any because it's a personal choice. Not everybody finds the same type of music relaxing. That being said, many of my patients have found these to be of benefit. Lower-frequency sound (1–4 hertz) is in the *delta* range and creates a state in the brain similar to meditation or deep sleep. Higher frequencies (14–30 hertz) are in the *alpha* range, which help with concentration and alertness.

Dr. Porges, creator of the polyvagal theory, also invented a tool using filtered music called the Safe and Sound Protocol, which can help people with anxiety and behaviors. I've had some experience with it helping people come out of a stuck high-activation and also low-activation nervous system. He created it to help young people with autism, but as research is ongoing, there might be other conditions that consistently improve.

LET'S PRACTICE—PLAYLISTS

Imagine that you're in the high-activation, restless stress response. Your body is tense, agitated. Your mind is racing. What kind of music would help you decompress? Is there something that you could move to, to release the tension in your muscles? It doesn't have to be a dance—rocking, swaying, or moving your hands around is enough.

Now, imagine that you are in a low-activation, listless stress response. Your body feels heavy and doesn't want to move. Your mind feels numb. What kind of music could help you activate a bit? Even moving your head, a hand, or a hip is a good start.

One thing I recommend is creating a *polyvagal playlist*—music suitable for these states.

Most people want something with high energy when their body is agitated. But you have to be careful not to tip it into a full-on panic. So, the music might be upbeat, rather than loud. Check in with your body to determine how fast the rhythm should be. If it's really frantic, that might make the activation state worse (or it might feel just right). The point is to let go of the tension your muscles hold.

When the body is feeling low energy, the music that resonates is typically quieter and slower. But you don't want it to be so mellow that you worsen a sense of dissociation. The goal is to entice you to move, just a little. Humming quietly, tapping a foot, is sufficient to shift the nervous system in the direction toward movement.

I encourage you to consider making these playlists, keep them updated, and use them when one of these nervous system states kicks in.

Tingles

Autonomous sensory meridian response (ASMR) is a pleasant tingling sensation in the upper body. People experience this feeling through sensory input, typically something they are hearing or seeing. Words that come to mind when I think of the feeling are *delicious, sweet,* or *tingly*. There are many YouTube or TikTok videos intending to create this feeling, but it lands differently in every nervous system. What evokes the sensation in one person doesn't necessarily work for another.

For me, gentle whispered voices or rustling leaves cause ASMR. It also helps when the video background is somewhere in nature. Or being in a library, hearing soft speaking and pages turning from someone reading. For me, ASMR feels like bubbles at the back of my head.

ASMR sensation is a *glimmer* for many people. If a trigger creates the trauma response in the body, the kinds of sensory inputs that create ASMR are the opposite. Some examples that can be heard through audio or video include pouring tea, brushing long hair, blowing on dandelion fluff, or the crinkle of parchment paper.

Mindful attention to a task can create the ASMR experience. The next time that you comb your hair, cook a meal, or write with a pencil—pay attention to the sound that you make. Does it feel delicious somewhere in your body? When researchers do imaging studies on the brain to see what lights up during ASMR, it's the same parts when we get goosebumps.

I don't recommend meditation early in trauma work to everyone. When you let the mind wander during a trauma response, it doesn't always go to safe places. But mindfulness differs from meditation because it simply brings you to the present moment. Experiencing ASMR is a way to be grounded in the moment while in a calm body. That is exactly what heals a traumatized nervous system reflex.

Some people choose to create a small kit where they could access tools that could recalibrate their nervous system when they're feeling stuck in a trauma response. Could you include a piece of soft fabric that you could brush, or hold up to your ear? Or a pendant on a chain that you could move back and forth? You can also take something solid in your kit and tap it, which can produce ASMR. Or click a pen. It's about noticing what feels good in your body.

Sound

Noise can be a trauma trigger. The word *misophonia* relates to people who can't listen to certain sounds: especially chewing, sniffling, or loud breathing. The universally disliked "nails on a chalkboard." It creates intense anger, disgust, and the high activation fight-or-flight system.

I recommend that my patients try humming when they find themselves triggered by a sound. A longer exhale activates the calm nervous system. Vocalizations vibrate the lungs and the pleural sac around them. Just behind this is your vagus nerve. When you hum and vibrate your vagus nerve, it can help regulate your nervous system by stimulating the parasympathetic (calm) response.

Any noise can be calming. It can also be a pleasant distraction when you're feeling triggered by a memory or experience, when you're trying to relax your body and get to sleep, or when your mind is racing with catastrophic thinking. Sounds that tend to be the most helpful come from nature, like raindrops or ocean waves or reeds. Other people prefer instrumental music or chanting.

White noises are even, like static (a radio or television without a station). There are sounds named by colors—*pink noise* is the deeper sounds like pounding rain, heartbeats, or wind tunnels. *Brown noise* is deeper still—a drumming waterfall or rumbling thunder. *Green noise* has both the high- and low-frequency sounds filtered out, which is used mostly for blocking out other noises, so it can be helpful in the background to focus. There are other colors of noise, but less likely to be calming (*blue noise*, for example, is a high-pitched hissing).

Vision

Viewing a beautiful or interesting scene can be a pleasant distraction and allow for mindful presence in a moment. But there's more that the eyes can do to shift the nervous system into a calm state.

There are two therapies that use back-and-forth (like a tennis match) eye motion. EMDR has it right in the title: Eye Movement Desensitization and Reprocessing. Accelerated Resolution Therapy (ART) is a faster version of this method. By moving the eyes from side to side, it helps the brain create a window where we can change memories. There are theories on how this works, but no confirmed evidence. The most transformative work I've done in trauma processing has been through ART.

The high-activation nervous system is in charge of peripheral vision (I would guess this developed through scanning for danger). Many people have assumed the opposite, that it's the laser focus of central vision that's involved in the fight-or-flight response.

LET'S PRACTICE—VERGENCE

We create flexibility through focusing on something close and then looking far away. Going back and forth is *vergence*—we use this in a trauma therapy technique called *Brainspotting*.

Changing your perspective can literally bring out the calmer, low-activation nervous system.

With the head facing forward, hold something in front of your face. It could be a pen, a fork, or a toothbrush—something that doesn't make you create a story in your mind.

Focus your eyes on the object and breathe five cycles.

Now, direct your gaze behind the object at the farthest point in the room. Breathe five times.

Now let your view alternate back and forth between these two viewpoints. How do you feel?

Fawn

Fawning is a term that's sometimes associated with trauma. Some people say it's part of the low-activation nervous system.

A person who fawns is people-pleasing, trying to appease others to avoid making them mad. I don't think of this as a trauma response per se, which are more subconscious reflexes or nervous system states. Fawning is more a learned behavior that helped at an earlier stage (especially when you couldn't escape the danger). Learning boundaries, trusting your gut instinct, and standing up for yourself are things that need to be practiced.

Let's try a simple eye movement exercise that we use (a modified version of) in advanced ART around this response.

LET'S PRACTICE—THE CIRCUS

Think of a belief you'd like to shift related to control or power. Something like "Things don't work out for me," or "I'm not good enough."

Now, record the following words on your phone or other device so that you can listen to them while your eyes are busy. I recorded this audio exercise on the YouTube channel at the QR code for the moderntrauma.com website (see page xviii).

Moving your eyes from side to side, imagine you're entering a circus. You have change in your pocket, and the entrance fee is a quarter, so you drop the change into a slot. A friendly person in a bright blue wig behind the counter waves you through.

The first thing we visit is the house of mirrors. You walk in and notice distortion of your body. It's taller, then it's shorter. It's wider, then it's narrower. It contorts in different directions because of the mirror. The last mirror is backlit with a screen that asks you to put another quarter in the slot. Then, it writes, "What's the perfect way to see yourself?" You put the change into the machine and it whirs, lights spin above you, and the mirror reveals your exact body.

Next stop is the acrobats, where you put more change in the entrance gate. You watch the trapeze artists flying above you through the air and landing safely on tall platforms. A pair of athletes balance each other easily using one arm, changing positions with incredible strength. People fly from a trampoline, flipping gracefully onto a mat. A voice says overhead, "Who else is trying as hard as they can?" and a spotlight illuminates your head. Applause breaks out in the crowd just as enthusiastically as for the performers.

The last stop is the fortune teller, who wears garish pink makeup and long fingernails. This time, you put the change on her table next to a glowing crystal ball. She moves her hands slowly over the ball, while fog fills the room. When the mist clears, you can see the future you always dreamed about reflected on the ball. The fortune teller smiles at you through her gauze scarves.

You leave the circus feeling satisfied and confident. As you leave, your posture has changed.

Change

Part of what's effective in this exercise is the word *change*. You may not have noticed it. In ART, the creator Laney Rosenzweig uses a lot of wordplay. This is one language of the subconscious mind.

If the circus image is not one that you prefer, how else could you conceive of holding "change"—imagine a different, more pleasing scenario.

Could you put it into the slots that let you play video games where you get to win at different tasks? Could you put the coins into lockers that have vibrant images or special objects inside? Could you put it into a time machine that lets you observe the past and the future with different colors of lens (not everyone wants rose-colored glasses)?

What change would you like to see? To hear?

Every time you hear the jingle of coins in your pocket, this might be a new *glimmer*.

CHAPTER 17

Create

This chapter is about how trauma moves through the body. When you're stuck in a high-activation, sympathetic nervous system response, your body wants to fight off or run away (flight) from the danger. So, it sends a lot of energy to your muscles. Any movement can help release some of this stored tension.

But creativity and playfulness can also help you move toward a calmer nervous system. Smaller amounts of activity might be more available to you if you are in the freeze state, so pay attention to what feels possible and what needs shifting. All of this is a menu, where you decide what to sample.

Many practices in this chapter come from my work in refugee communities and my reading about Indigenous healing practices. Psychotherapies were created with the white experience and white body in mind, so body-based (somatic) and creative practices might be more acceptable and effective for people with varied experiences or a different culture. I've mentioned Resmaa Menakem's work in *Somatic Abolitionism*—embodied antiracist practices—these are worth exploring.

Moving Up the Ladder

Deb Dana describes the polyvagal ladder where freezing or shutting down is at the bottom of the ladder, and you move through a higher activation in order to get to the calm and connected state. In polyvagal language, dorsal vagal is the bottom, sympathetic is the middle, and ventral vagal is the top of the ladder.

POLYVAGAL
LADDER

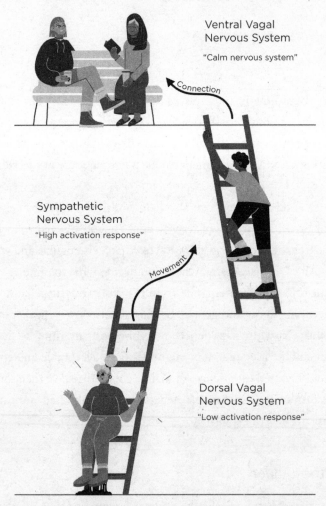

Ventral Vagal
Nervous System

"Calm nervous system"

Connection

Sympathetic
Nervous System

"High activation response"

Movement

Dorsal Vagal
Nervous System

"Low activation response"

Credit: Deb Dana, Dr. Stephen Porges

If we start (feeling stuck) at the bottom of the ladder, then creativity and expression provide enough movement to begin the journey up. What gets us unstuck is movement. What gets us to calm is connection.

Express Yourself

Trauma can leave us unable to notice how we feel, because our thinking brain goes offline during an intense trauma response. There are other ways of expressing feelings without stating them. Getting the tone across in a poem. Telling a story with meaning. Singing a song that evokes the same emotion.

An unexpected trauma therapy is through the company DE-CRUIT. It's a variation of the word *recruit*, because it's designed for military veterans who suffer from PTSD. People serving in the military have a higher proportion of ACEs (adverse childhood experiences). So, the PTSD from combat or injury is often layered on top of complex trauma (multiple kinds of stressful events over different occasions). DE-CRUIT teaches Shakespearean monologues that share an emotional response when the person can't find words. The script shows them how to express it. Performance art, theater in this case, allows people to reenact an emotion or event with distance. It doesn't feel as personal if you're playing a character.

Another practice that helps a person express how they feel about system-level trauma is Theater of the Oppressed. Systemic traumas include racism, sexism, classism—the "isms" and more (homophobia, fat phobia).

In this theater production, the audience jumps into the show. They can either shout suggestions at the actors or they can substitute for a person onstage and enact their idea. This will typically happen around solving social problems or dealing with a person who's being mistreated. This sense of control over the situation creates a powerful reenactment of a trauma experience with lots of support. The word for this feeling of control is *agency*.

Silly

Acting a certain way changes your nervous system. The movie *Patch Adams* is based on a real physician who uses humor to create a bond with patients. He began clowning around, being silly to get a laugh, on the wards as a med student. He soon realized that the medical system wasn't always effective at helping people with mental health problems. Now, he clowns with a purpose, visiting communities with low resources and bringing infectious joy. I went on one of his group visits to Mexico City in early 2020, just before the COVID-19 pandemic, where I studied humanitarian clowning. Yes, that's a thing. I have a red leather nose to prove it. We visited many people, including those in prisons, facilities for severely disabled persons, and a hospital.

Laughter, like yawning, can be infectious. The sound of it activates the calm nervous system. Especially when people in authority (a doctor like Patch or me) can lighten up a space with laughter, vulnerability, and humility—we create the conditions for a person to feel safer. Laughter also creates long exhales, and the vibration against your chest soothes the vagus nerve.

Laughter is medicine.

LET'S PRACTICE—THE PEAK

Imagine yourself watching a movie of a recent event that was distressing. It could be about spilling a drink, a minor injury, or forgetting something. Try not to make the story too emotional.

Imagine watching a short movie of this story in your mind. You could also write it out so that it takes less than one page.

As we imagine this video or short story, we're going to let it show up the way writers develop the plot of a novel. (Hint: The tension shows up in the middle.) For those familiar with a bell curve, it peaks at the halfway point.

Fill in the details from the beginning, when tension slowly builds up and toward the end when everything has settled down. Make sure that the ending brings everything back to a calm place, both emotionally and physically.

One therapy that uses this kind of technique is the Counting Method, where you would count out loud to 100 while imagining something uncomfortable. You want to time the story in a similar way, so the distressing emotions and situations happen around the numbers 50 to 60. By the time you get to 90, any emotion and fear settle out of the story.

Games

Fascinating research has come out in the last few years about the video game *Tetris*. In one study, researchers exposed subjects to a horror movie, but when reactivating the memory four days later, they were asked to either play *Tetris* or a word game. Compared to the control group, both activities took away the flashbacks related to the movie.

After this came out, people researched *Tetris* in another study, asking subjects to write a story about a traumatic event. Without talking about it, they tore up the piece of paper and then played the video game. Because these people were inpatients in the hospital, they were studied for quite a while and did the intervention more than once. For the memories that they wrote and associated with the video game, flashbacks about those events improved drastically.

The theory is that the same part of the brain that deals with visuospatial information is needed for both the flashbacks and the game, so it interferes with the memory and rewrites on top of it. Sadly, the research wasn't consistent, because when they had people play *Tetris* in the emergency room after a car crash, intrusive memories improved only in the short term. All the other symptoms of PTSD, that high-activation nervous system and the alarm bells going off, persisted. And the effects didn't last when they checked in with the subjects one month later.

All of this is good news, because it means that people are getting creative in how they research PTSD. Since we don't have effective medication, we have to rely on neurobiology. I'm sure pharmaceutical companies search for the magic elixir, but so much of the trauma response happens in a relationship and in a community, which doesn't have a quick fix.

Images

Creating together in a community can be part of the healing process for many people. At our refugee clinic in Calgary, there's an art therapy group running for many years for people with trauma responses. By drawing or making shapes about emotions and situations, it allows people to feel mastery over the problem while also changing it in a way they prefer. When they're able to avoid talking about it, this gives them a safer distance from the traumatic content.

The subconscious mind, where reflex trauma responses occur, doesn't use the language of words. It uses the language of imagery and metaphor. So, it makes sense that art can be healing. It doesn't have to be painting—ceramics and sculpture would work too.

Expressing how something feels without using words is a powerful thing to do. I learned an exercise from a group from the Scottish community of Findhorn that I think would be useful for people dealing with stress and trauma.

LET'S PRACTICE—QUADRANTS

This exercise requires paper and something to write with, or a drawing app on a tablet. But, of course, you could get as creative and colorful as you like.

Take the rectangular-shaped page and divide it into four boxes. In the first box, draw a picture of your current state. This could be your identity, your location, your profession, or your emotions.

In the next box, draw how you would like to be in the future. These drawings don't have to be artistic. Try to do them in under a minute or two so you don't put any pressure on yourself. They can also be metaphors instead of an image, like a cloud or a lightbulb or a tree.

In the third box, draw an image or metaphor of something that is causing an obstruction. What is in your way to get from here to there (from box 1 to 2)?

In the last box, draw a combination of the second and third boxes. They could merge, they could be in a battle, they could be overlapping. How can you combine these two ideas so that they become singular?

What have you learned about your obstacle that you might not have thought of if you were using words? Does making the drawing tell you something new?

When I practiced this exercise, my obstruction was a box that "contained" me. It was constricting. Then my solution was to turn the square (solid box) into a screen (frame). I noticed that the solution helped me free up new possibilities—helped create the mental flexibility that's so essential to healing and growing.

Music

Music therapy is an intensely healing practice. A few years ago, a group of us were talking about ways that healing can happen outside of traditional medicine. We ended up creating a cooperative.

A key member of our team is Tiffany Sparrow, a music therapist who did graduate work in ethnomusicology (how different cultures incorporate music for healing). She accommodated all the different languages and nationalities that came to our program, finding songs from each culture that made people feel sentimental and connected.

Tiffany and I designed the four-week intervention deliberately. Our first session was an invitation where we met everybody, so she created a lovely little round about "being welcome here." The second session was about a high-activation response, so she and Emma Harding (singing teacher) created an energetic program that would help release tension. The third session was for a low-activation response, so it was more gentle and soothing but still engaged. The last session was about gratitude. These practices have a lot of science behind them, but that's not necessarily something that the participants had to think about. They just showed up to do exercises with their breath, sing some pleasant songs, and meet new people.

Music therapy can shift traumatic responses because there are so many ways to express yourself. The sound of the music. Lyrics and emotional tone. When Tiffany worked in a hospital, she used to write songs with people dying in the palliative care ward. I honestly can't think of anything more meaningful than that. And you certainly can't make a pill to heal in quite the same way.

When I struggled in medical school, and during other times in my life where I had big emotions, I enjoyed writing poetry. Some people do this with rap lyrics. Others might recite spoken word. These are ways to express how we're feeling without having to make it confessional or conversational.

Move

As these small amounts of activity move us up the polyvagal ladder, we can turn our attention to more intentional movement practices.

Starting off gently, an easy walk is a practice that I recommend to people who feel that they can physically do it. Being in nature, especially with a pet or on an outdoor pathway with a nice view, is beneficial for the nervous system.

During the COVID-19 pandemic, I discovered an app that I really enjoyed called The Conqueror. The price might not be accessible to all—you could design one on your own using Google Maps. The app allows you to pick the place where you'll pretend to walk. So far, I have "climbed" Everest from base camp and Mount Fuji in Japan, then "hiked" the Camino de Santiago in Spain and the Ring of Kerry in Ireland. Every day that you walk, you enter the distance that you did into the app. Then, it moves your little avatar along the pathway. It sends you postcards along the journey of sites you would have seen, and you can use the Google "street view" function to see each location. In the winter, I decided to "go" to a sunny beach in France. This would be an easy thing to do if you pull up any of these destinations on a Google Map and keep the tab open in your browser. Move the pointer along for every walk that you take and have a look around.

Beyond walking (for people who have the energy to do it), I always recommend aerobic exercise that gets your heart rate up to let go of the sympathetic tone that builds in your body. This will be different for each person, but my favorite recommendations include dance programs or martial arts. When you are doing an activity in a group where everybody moves in synchrony, the chemicals in your brain allow a deeper relaxation response. So, not only do you get the benefit of your muscle tone being released, you get this extra comfort of being a literal part of a movement.

Movement helps heal a stressed body, because you get the benefits of releasing the muscle tone without having the constant danger signals of fight-or-flight. This can help reprogram the body to associate a pounding heart, sweating, and muscle contraction with something enjoyable rather than something scary.

adrienne maree brown speaks to systemic trauma issues and *somatic practices*. The organization Generative Somatics works at the intersection of movement, justice, and oppression. It's not just about movement, but the social conditions in which we live. Because so much trauma is political, creative expression and movement are ways to express and align with deeper transformation practices.

One of the most effective forms of treating trauma is *neurofeedback*, where the therapist or researcher attaches electrodes to your skull to measure your brain waves. When your brain waves are calm, it signals your body to let you know that you're on track. These creative tools can work in the same way—to associate a sense of calm to your activities. When you pair this with the trauma memories or responses—your brain creates new associations. New pathways.

CHAPTER 18

Havening

Human bodies evolved with resources that heal stress and trauma. As we enhance our understanding of the mind-body connection, we can craft new strategies.

Havening Techniques™ is one of my favorite skills to teach people. It's simple. It's effective. And, unlike medicine's chemical solutions, there are no side effects. It creates a shift in brain waves that calms the mind. I saw it firsthand, with a video of my brain waves changing on a screen during training.

When I heard about Havening, I was skeptical. It seemed too easy. The Ruden brothers (a doctor and a dentist) who invented the technique hadn't done the level of research I'm used to. Generally, new medical treatments go through randomized controlled trials (RCT)—evidence that's the highest level of rigor. In these, there's a placebo (control group with no intervention) or "gold standard" (the best treatment so far) measured against a new intervention, with random assignments for each group. While the Ruden brothers examined the research to learn which touch technique was effective, researchers haven't done many RCT yet. It's still early days, though.

Havening touch causes a higher percentage of slow, calm brain waves. You can use it as self-touch, so you can do it on your own, anywhere and anytime.

There's an accompanying video to this practice on the website linked to the QR code on page xviii.

The premise of the Havening Techniques is there are many things a human can do to create delta waves in the brain. Our brain, like our heart, is full of electricity. For the brain, we measure it with an EEG (electroencephalogram) and for the heart, it's an ECG (electrocardiogram). It's ironic when physicians dismiss energy medicine because we already look at these energy levels for evidence of health. Practitioners call these energy tools *psychosensory techniques*.

Delta waves are naturally calming; we would get them when we're winding down at the end of a day or in a deep sleep. Most of the time, when delta waves dominate, other waves (like gamma, which relate to thinking and alertness) will go down. I watched this in real time when I learned the techniques.

This change occurred while I was thinking about the scariest thing that's ever happened to me. Now, that memory has changed forever.

In April 2015, I was working with a medical school in Nepal. I was in my apartment in Patan, in the Kathmandu Valley, when an earthquake hit. Reading a 7.8 on the Richter scale, it was massive. The building shook so hard that I could hear the cracks breaking through the wall. When I ran down the stairs, it was like the tile steps had liquefied and were moving in every direction. It was surreal to watch objects lose their solid properties and crumble. Talk about watching energy shift.

I was terrified.

The surrounding buildings were coming down with booming sounds. One after another, I heard the crashes of collapse. Vibrations pounded through every bone of my body. Racing as fast as I could down the stairs, I pulled open the heavy wooden doors into the courtyard. They were sticking because the building was shaking so much and the warped door frame didn't fit properly anymore. When I finally got the door open, after a few seconds that seemed to stretch for hours (this is normal during a trauma), I could see the courtyard was full of bricks and cement dust. More was coming down in what looked like a landslide. Tearful, coughing—I slammed the door shut, looking around for somewhere safe. There was a heavy table in the lobby next to the shared washing machine. I dove under it and hung onto the legs. It bounced as the floor shook; I could tell my knees were getting banged up on the slate. What felt like two hours was less than two minutes in reality. But reality was messed up. There's a painting by Salvador Dalí where a watch is melting and dripping off a table—that's how the world seemed to me. Surreal. Scary. Shocking.

After the first earthquake, I ran back upstairs for my laptop to call my parents. All I wanted was for them to rescue me—to tell me everything would be okay. Even though it was three o'clock in the morning in Canada, my mom picked up the Skype call. She walked me through a website about how to survive an earthquake. My dad told me in soft, reassuring tones that I was safe. I could viscerally feel my nervous system calming down; my heart didn't pound so hard and I wasn't sweating anymore. After that call, my frantic mind could focus on the next steps. Including facing the massive aftershocks, then checking on the hospital staff, who rescued the injured. Many Nepali physician colleagues slept in the hospital, despite the deep crevices in the walls, to serve their communities. It was inspiring, but terrifying.

If you want to hear my story, and the devastating impact on locals, check out my TEDx Talk "Journey from Hero to Humility" and our nonprofit site Global Familymed Foundation where you can support the Patan training hospital—Patan Academy of Health Sciences (PAHS).

The tragedy lived out loud in my brain until three years later, when I learned about Havening and reprogrammed those same memories.

The premise of Havening came from researchers who attached EEG monitors while inviting participants to perform a series of simple activities. They could see which actions increased calm delta brain waves.

Researchers discovered one of the ways that the body knows how to heal itself. The three areas of the body that created the most delta waves (with a gentle brushing movement of the opposite hand) are the ones we already use to soothe.

HAVENING TOUCH

Palm Havening	Arm Havening	Face Havening
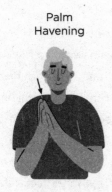	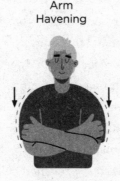	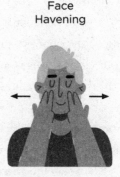

Credit: Dr. Ronald Ruden

We create delta waves by brushing our fingertips across the palm of our opposite hand. I believe Havening works best in a single direction (the same way a dog or cat prefers petting in the direction of their fur).

Contact your hands with your palms together. Slowly drag one hand downward until it reaches the crease of your wrist, gently brushing your fingertips across your other palm. Move back to the starting position and do the same thing with your opposite hand.

We learned that this area of the body creates five times the delta waves compared to a resting state. What's remarkable is it seems the body organically knows this. People may wring their hands when they're stressed. We hold hands with somebody we care about, including at a time when they are upset and need reassurance. If our hands get sweaty because we're anxious, we wipe them on something. These actions would naturally create delta waves, but until the researchers studied this, we didn't understand the physiology behind the response.

Two other areas of the body create delta waves with similar movements. Reach across to touch your palm against your opposite shoulder, then brush downward toward your elbow. The amount of pressure is as if you were petting an animal. It's not a massage and it's not a light tickle. Something in between. It doesn't need to be against skin; clothing doesn't prevent the response.

If you reach across your body with both arms until each hand is resting on the opposite shoulder and then move your palms downward toward your elbows, this is the technique that Dr. Kate Truitt, one of my teachers, calls the "moving hug." This makes sense, too—we naturally hug someone who's upset to help them feel better. So, providing some of the same sensation, even to ourselves, should be calming. Being patted on the shoulder is a sign of support between humans.

The area of the body that creates the most delta waves is on the face—the research showed it was up to ninety times compared to sleeping. Starting from the middle, brushing gently with two fingers on either side of your nose, swipe across your cheekbone toward the temples, moving lightly across your skin. Next, start from the middle again and brush across your forehead or eyebrows. All three areas create a large amount of delta wave brain activity.

While this isn't something that another human might do as an adult, many mothers instinctively do this with their babies. Lightly touching the infant's face, brushing their fingertips across their forehead. And it's something that we naturally do when we cry; we wipe our hands across our cheekbones to wipe our tears.

You can see how the three areas where the Havening Techniques take place are all areas where we have an instinct to self-soothe.

The researchers also discovered delta activity increased from moving the eyes side to side, a method used in many therapies, including EMDR and ART.

When I learned these techniques and experienced a practice session, the trainer attached an EEG electrode to my forehead. While my teacher walked me through the Havening protocols, they projected my brain waves on a screen behind me. The delta waves doubled while agitated gamma waves decreased.

During the session, I recalled the entire sequence of my experience of the earthquakes in Nepal. The teacher helped me pair new emotions and physical sensations with the memory. These have been permanent changes.

When you access a memory, it's a time when you can change it. We
store traumatic memory associations in our amygdalas instead of the hippocampus. Think of the amygdalas as a mailbox with a red flag on it that
gets threatening postcards with unpleasant images. Think of the hippocampus as a filing cabinet that integrates other memories, written like stories
where you could easily speak about the event. The traumatic messages in
the mailbox might have just a couple of images on the postcard, related to
the context of what happened. These memories are often difficult to tell as
a cohesive story. They're fragments of images and scenarios, sounds and
tastes, sensations like a rolling in the gut or pounding in the chest.

When we access traumatic memories, there's a 48- to 72-hour window
where we can change them. The Havening Techniques create some of
those possibilities. This is a phenomenon called *neuroplasticity*. Your brain
comprises over eighty billion neurons, special cells of the central nervous
system (brain and spinal cord), and peripheral nervous system (through
muscles and internal organs). In the brain, neural connections create patterned movements, coordinated effort, store memories, and allow critical
thinking. We can rewire many areas of the brain. After a trauma, the brain
visits those same pathways toward threatening past events. These are experienced in the present moment as flashbacks or triggers.

The best way to change this pattern is to provide a new pathway. Accessing the memory, pairing it with new physical symptoms and different emotions, can be part of the rewiring. When you do it while your body creates
extra delta waves, you maintain a restful nervous system so you can stay in
a calm body even while accessing traumatic material.

The key is staying in a calm body.

When we reexperience these traumatic memories, the body tends to go
into (sympathetic) overactivity or (dorsal vagal) shutdown. When we're able
to reexperience aspects of the danger while in a calm (ventral vagal) body,

this is where neuroplasticity becomes possible. We can change the pathways of trauma responses when we have mental flexibility. Neuroplasticity allows us to reprogram those memories in a way we'd prefer.

We can give this a try, if you like. Remember, there's a recording on the book's website (through the QR code; see page xviii), if you want to listen and use both hands. There's also a video of a longer Havening session.

LET'S PRACTICE—SELF-HAVENING

Imagine a scenario that's not traumatic, because we don't want you practicing something alone that would cause a *flood* (too many emotions) or a *freeze* (emotional numbing) reaction.

Picture the context when this scenario happened. It should be something that was irritating, but not much more activating than that. Who was around? Was it indoors or outdoors? What time of day? How did you feel at the time? Do you remember the emotions that you had? Any physical sensations?

Give this memory a rating. In psychology, we would say SUDS, which stands for *subjective unit of distress scale*. Subjective, because you get to decide. Everybody has different reactions after they've experienced similar events. A unit of distress is a method that we can measure how much something bothers you. So, a zero on the scale would be something that doesn't bother you whatsoever. But a 10 would be the most distressing thing you could imagine. What would you give this memory as a SUDS number? If it's higher than 4, it's probably better to practice with something less activating.

Now, we are going to do Havening to provide new physical symptoms and emotions to associate with that memory.

Slowly brush your palms, fingertips dragging gently down each hand.

Let's imagine going for a walk in the jungle. This isn't a place where we're going to encounter anything threatening, like spiders or snakes. You get to choose animals you'd want to encounter. Imagine some birds in the trees. What sounds are they making? What colors are they?

What other sounds do you hear in the jungle? Maybe there's the grunting of monkeys playing in the canopy overhead or croaking of frogs in a nearby pond.

Look around you and notice three different colors. I bet one of them is green? Now, notice two distinct smells.

Start applying a Havening touch to your arms, brushing from your shoulders down toward your elbows in a moving hug. Go slowly, maybe three to five seconds for each movement.

Walk toward a tree and notice cute, fuzzy caterpillars crawling up and down. Count eight of them and then keep walking. Notice the soft feeling of leaves underfoot.

There's a treehouse in the jungle. It can be as high as you prefer, maybe only a couple of feet off the ground or perhaps high in the treetops. There's a sturdy ladder welcoming you. Climb up, counting the rungs. Picture the movement of each leg pushing to propel yourself upward.

Your head pops into the treehouse first, and the ladder continues until your whole body is inside. Slide a little trap door closed so there's nothing to fall through. Look around, noticing some beanbag chairs on the floor or a futon. There's also a basket of fresh fruit on a table. Go over to the basket and notice three fruits that are inside. You may choose to pick one of them up, to smell or bite.

Continue by brushing your face. Move your fingers from the midline across your cheekbones, your forehead, and your eyebrows.

Looking at the tropical sky, notice that the sun is setting. Describe the colors that bloom across the sky and reflect in the clouds. There's a monkey hanging by its tail outside the window of the treehouse. The monkey chatters, holding a banana in its hand. You wonder if it's a banana from your fruit bowl and burst out laughing.

When you're done, take your time and rest your hands in your lap. Take a few deep breaths. Check in with your body. Did the activation that was created from thinking back to the memory come up again? When you think of the same event, what is your SUDS number now?

CHAPTER 19

Tapping

I first heard about the Tapping technique through physicians at a youth health clinic. They used it with the adolescents who had incredibly stressful lives, with beneficial effects. They recommended a place where I could learn, but I really didn't know what I was getting into until I arrived for the weekend training in Washington State.

Tapping, also called Emotional Freedom Techniques (EFT), is based on ancient technology. Acupuncture is part of Traditional Chinese Medicine (TCM), where practitioners stick tiny needles into your skin along energy (chi or qi) lines, the meridians. In my professional experience, I've seen it help with chronic pain, fertility, and many other well-researched illnesses. But until then, I'd never heard of this used in the context of emotions.

The first related practice that developed from acupuncture was Thought Field Therapy (TFT). When I studied this technique, each emotion had a different sequence to remember. One sequence for grief, another for fear, yet another for anger. It quickly gets overwhelming.

EFT uses the most intense points of energy for these emotions and puts it into a single sequence. The person who invented it was a minister and coach; many people who practice it aren't regulated mental health providers (which makes me a bit nervous in the context of trauma). They've learned to coach people through the sequence.

It seems the body naturally dials emotions down with these techniques. The evidence is mounting that it's effective for emotional regulation, even cravings and the symptoms of traumatic reflex responses. It takes practice to build muscle memory, but after two or three sessions, most people have the pattern down.

I think of it as acupressure, using touch instead of needles. So, EFT is *self-acupressure*, designed to dial the volume down on emotional experiences. Emotions don't have to be labeled as good or bad, but if they feel stuck or too intense, they can cause unnecessary suffering.

HERE'S AN EXAMPLE

Bridges always frighten Daria. When she's in a car that goes over a river or a valley, as soon as the wheels leave the road attached to the earth, her heart drops into her stomach. She has a memory of her older brother teasing her—the other kids ran across the railway bridge, but her own feet froze at the edge. She remembers stumbling across the tracks, imagining she could hear the train whistle. Living in the Bay Area doesn't help. Daria goes over a bridge more often than she'd like. Worries consume her mind about what would happen if an earthquake hit while she's over the water. She dreams about these terrors, waking up sweaty and tearful.

The association of an object or context that causes emotions to show up after a reminder of an event is a *conditioned response*. The word *conditioned* means that there is a pairing of the emotion and the trigger. This works like a feedback loop. Feedback means that every time it happens, the association and emotion intensify. And loop means that you feel trapped, unable to escape this response. Here's where EFT comes in, by breaking the loop.

You can watch a video introduction of the practice from the QR code on page xviii.

The sequence starts by tapping along the side of your hand. We call this the *setup point*. Between the base of your smallest finger and the crease of your wrist, on the far side of your hand, is where we begin the practice. You can tap this area with all fingers, or your palm, of your other hand. As you do that, you repeat the setup phrase.

TAPPING EFT

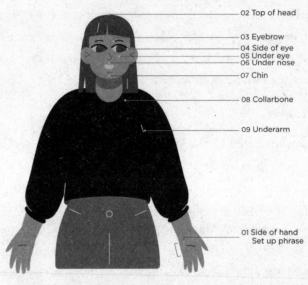

02 Top of head

03 Eyebrow
04 Side of eye
05 Under eye
06 Under nose
07 Chin

08 Collarbone

09 Underarm

01 Side of hand
Set up phrase

Credit: Gary Craig

Once this step is over, continue the rest of the sequence. I tap on each of the areas five to seven times, but I've seen people do it much longer, thirty or more times. There doesn't seem to be a consensus on the best way to do it. I use a slow pace, but some instructors go faster, so again, I don't think that there's a single way to do it. Notice what feels best for you.

Tap your head with two fingers of each hand. One hand works if that's what's accessible to you. In fact, you can imagine the movements and those areas of your brain will light up.

Start at the top of your head, move to your inner eyebrow, then your temple area, to your cheekbone right underneath the center of your eye, then change to one hand between your nose and upper lip, then between your lower lip and chin. Go back to both hands, where your collarbones meet your breastbone (in medical terms, we would say the clavicles connect to the sternum). This place is harder to landmark because you need to find the knobs where the collarbones finish in the midline; line up your second fingers with those bony prominences, and then the rest of your fingers tap vertically along either side of your breastbone. The last place is directly under your armpit, where a bra line would be on a person who wears one. You can move your arm outward like a chicken wing and use the top of your hand to tap in the area. Or, if it works for your body, you can wrap your arms across your front to tap on your opposite side with your fingertips.

Most people who teach EFT have a slightly different sequence, and I've trained with three different instructors so far, so I combine all of their techniques in my demonstrations to patients. Just like the other somatic techniques, I don't recommend using a traumatic memory when you're practicing this on your own. But that doesn't mean that we can't work on the symptoms of trauma in the present moment.

Emotional pain and physical pain are simply messages between the body and the brain. You can turn the volume dial down on the message while still paying attention to it and work on the causes of the message or what it's telling you. Tapping can be a tool to work on the symptoms from previous trauma, to help shift our nervous systems out of too much overactivity or underactivity. In fact, there is enough research on this method that it's considered an evidence-based treatment for PTSD.

Accessing distressing emotions while you tap changes your nervous system so that signals don't overwhelm. Over time, the brain rewires so these emotions don't show up in such an intense way.

I recommend using a setup phrase introducing "There is" rather than "I am." It sounds similar, but it makes a significant difference in how our subconscious mind hears the message. When you say that you are an emotion, you're telling your brain that you identify with it. That it belongs to you. That you are attached to this feeling. When you provide some distance, normalize the emotion as something that we all experience as humans, and you are just experiencing a portion at this moment, the subconscious mind doesn't identify as much.

Let's do a few sequences to show you what I mean.

LET'S PRACTICE—BASIC EFT

Tapping on the side of your hand, say the setup phrase three times:

"Even though there's a nervous feeling about learning how to tap, and I'm noticing there's a knot in my stomach, I completely accept all my feelings about this."

Say this line, or something that feels better for you with your own physical symptoms and perhaps a different emotion, three times out loud or in your mind.

Now go through the series of tapping points, saying "This nervous feeling," or the emotion you chose, at each position.

Take a couple of deep breaths when you're done and check in with your body to see if it feels any different after trying this technique.

I'll invite you to do a second round.

Pick something that everyone is familiar with but not triggering. If the following example doesn't work for you, please substitute a different emotion and situation. Something specific, especially if you can tie it to a recent event, works best.

We'll start with another version of the setup phrase, three times while tapping on the side of your hand.

"Even though there is this grief, with a hollow feeling in my chest. I notice it sometimes when I wish there was someone around. Right here, right now, I am safe."

After you've said this three times, move through the other points again. As you tap each area, you say "This grief," or any other emotion you chose to practice for the second round.

When I reach the collarbones, a very active point in acupressure (K-27), sometimes I say "I am safe" instead of naming the emotion again.

With Tapping, we also rate the intensity of emotion and physical sensations (before and after) using the SUDS numbers. That way, you can tell clearly if the feelings shift.

Rate your SUDS number from zero to ten before you start and then after you do a round. If using zero through ten isn't something that is easy to do around your emotions, try small, medium, or large. Or use a thermometer color chart. Or smile-to-frown face scales. We can choose different SUDS for cultural interpretations, for neurodivergence, and just for preferences. It's all subjective.

LET'S PRACTICE—THIS FEELING

Tapping the side of your hand, say the setup phrase three times:

"Even though there is sadness about being alone, this disconnected feeling, almost like feeling numb, I'd rate this feeling at a four out of ten. And even though there is sadness when I think about my friends that I haven't seen in a long time, I'm curious if this is something I could shift."

When you start the setup phrase with this language, at each of the tapping points, you would say something like "This alone feeling" or "This sadness."

Sometimes, when it's hard to name the emotion, here is a technique that works really well: "This blah feeling" or "This hot-and-cold feeling" or "This under-the-weather feeling."

After you've done one round, if it hasn't budged your SUDS number, consider doing a second round with the same feeling. Check in with your physical sensations to see if they are the same. Has the emotion shifted?

Try another round and see if you can get the SUDS number to zero, or at least less than two.

In this last session, we touched on one of the core developmental wounds that children possess. The pain of connection and the pain of solitude are intense, so we need to learn how to navigate them both safely as adults. Connection can feel unsatisfying, but when we don't have any at all, many people crave it.

EFT is more effective when you choose a specific event related to the emotion. Name a detail or two to evoke the memory. Then, you can see if the same emotion is still attached to it once you've done a sequence.

LET'S PRACTICE—CONTAIN IT

This is another version of the Container technique. It's used in many therapies other than EFT, including EMDR.

Imagine a container for your darkest memories, so that they no longer bother you. Is it a box or a rounder container? Is it metal, wood, or cardboard? How secure is the lid, and is there a lock? What color, size, age, shape, and weight is it?

Let's decide where to put it, maybe under the basement stairs at your parent's home. Maybe bury it somewhere. Whatever feels like the safest option.

Say the setup phrase three times, substituting these details that you just chose:

"Even though there is this container, filled with the things I'm still working on, made out of this material and about this heavy, this color, and placed in this area...right here, right now, I am safe."

Then, you would go through the sequence of all the other tapping points, and at each place name a characteristic of the container. At the collarbone points, I reinforce safety.

This Container technique is one of my favorites. I often ask if the container might hold shame, guilt, or fear. As we practiced, sometimes the container needs to be left at somebody else's home or another significant place where it's given back to the person who tried to give this emotion to you.

LET'S PRACTICE—SNEAK AWAY

The Sneaking Away technique is another EFT tool that I really enjoy. It's a reminder to the system to close the session, that the work of the day is over.

Tap the side of your hand with this phrase, then select one or two words along each tapping point:

"Even though I have done some work today, there is still much to do. I've made some headway, I can see progress, and I know there's more to be done. And even though I am proud of myself for the shifts that I managed today, I'm curious about how much more can be done."

"Some progress."

"Headway."

"Curious."

Use any of these words, or simply stick to one of them, as you tap the rest of the sequence.

There are dozens more techniques. But these are great ones to start with, demonstrating the power of the mind to change our memory storage.

There is one last point that I learned from one of my Tapping instructors, Dr. Craig Weiner, but it applies to most people who are trying to work through their trauma. We note resistance in Tapping when the SUDS number stays the same. Craig described three main reasons why there might be resistance to healing. I've confirmed these in my practice and will add a fourth.

1. A person's identity is entwined with their trauma. It's the main lens through which they see their experiences. It's how they define themselves as a human in the present moment. Often, Tapping might work on superficial aspects of the problem, but the foundational beliefs persist.
2. The person doesn't feel safe to let go of the issue. This could be because they don't feel comfortable in their relationship with their therapist or coach. They may be stuck in some emotional or physical danger. Or maybe they believe maintaining a level of emotion, especially something like anger or fear, keeps them safer.

3. There can be *secondary gain*, which means that they benefit somehow from the intense emotion. As a physician, the most common benefit that a person has for maintaining mental health symptoms is the label of disability, which helps keep support and care from family or professionals, staying off work, and additional financial assistance. It's one more reason I advocate for guaranteed income, so people can spend their time in how they choose, but people with disabilities can still have a reasonable quality of life.

4. *Survivor guilt* is common in my practice—feeling bad for having survived. A person who had to leave their family behind in a refugee camp. A sibling whose younger sister is not doing well. Especially working in addiction medicine, a person struggles to heal when most of their friends and sometimes family still suffer with substance use.

One of the most common books to learn EFT is *The Tapping Solution*. It uses a different technique than I describe here. It also endorses people working through their trauma, watching the entire movie of their childhood, on their own. The founder of EFT, Gary Craig, described a "personal peace procedure" where he recommends making a list of everything that's ever bothered you in your life and tapping through the list as you go. I'm hesitant to recommend this because it could unearth some deep wounds that might cause flooding or freezing. Those reactions are difficult to handle by yourself. Could you do most of these events? Absolutely. But trust your intuition if your gut instinct tells you it's going to be too much.

That's another opportunity to practice (re)learning how to trust our suppressed instincts.

What I like about *The Tapping Solution* is how it focuses not just on emotions about an event but also chronic pain, phobias, and cravings. While I haven't had the same level of success with my own patients, I have seen some benefits.

When I studied the more advanced techniques for Tapping, one that I really enjoyed was prompting "and that might mean..." or "I'm guessing it's because..." and letting your mind quickly fill in the blank.

Another useful advanced technique is to picture your younger self who went through something challenging, again not something too dangerous, but perhaps when you felt lonely or scared. You picture your younger self's hairstyle, what clothes they might have worn, and details about the room they'd be in. Then you, as an adult, would sit near this imaginary child in your mind and ask for their permission to tap the EFT sequence on them, to help them lower their emotions. It's a fantastic way to go back and heal our past wounded selves. Those Exiles.

The two phrases that I use the most in teaching and practicing EFT are both powerful for trauma:

"I deeply and completely accept myself..."
"Right here, right now, I am safe..."

Imagine how powerfully your life would change if you could believe that. Of course, you could start smaller if this feels incongruent or untrue.

"I can imagine a time when I accept myself."
"Right now, there is some safety, and I'm learning to access more."

An advantage of using EFT is that it helps you figure out your *limiting beliefs*. What are the things you believe about the world? Think scarcity compared to abundance. What are the things you believe about yourself? Whether you deserve success. Look for themes while you tap to see if you can figure out what those limiting beliefs are—and then tap on those.

Both Havening and Tapping are excellent techniques to teach children because the practices can help them regulate their own emotions. Plus, they're both simple to learn. They need to be taught by someone in a calm (ventral vagal) body, with a soothing voice and comforting emotions.

CHAPTER 20

Tremoring

Have you ever spent time with a dog? What about a horse? When these animals get stressed, they shake their entire body from top to tail. Then, they seem to move on.

It's not like there aren't anxious dogs—my companion, Fife, is a worrier. But I think such anxious tendencies come from conditioned responses or a predisposition; many animals can recover from a minor single event simply by shaking it off.

The human body can too.

Dr. David Berceli created Trauma (or Tension) Releasing Exercises (TRE) when he worked in countries coping with war. He has a doctorate in social work, but he's also a massage therapist (Rolfing), so he witnessed the trauma responses from both perspectives (the mind and the body).

Dr. Berceli noticed (described to us during training) that people who spontaneously shivered when they were afraid seemed to suffer less from PTSD after the event. Once, huddled in a bomb shelter in Lebanon, he recognized some people would tremor violently. It seemed to provide them relief, and they faced fewer trauma symptoms afterward. Based on these observations, he explored how he could teach this to the ones who don't naturally tremor.

This is an excellent illustration of how trauma is not the thing that happens to us, but our body's response. If our body can deal with the trauma at the moment and process it in real time, then it's less likely to get stuck in the body.

TRE isn't just intended for the immediate shock after a trauma; it can release muscle tension at any time. If your body is stuck in the high-activation sympathetic nervous system response, that means your muscles are always ready to run away or fight. This leaves them in constant tension, often causing pain in the limbs, back, or neck. TRE (more efficiently than other exercise) releases muscle tone and allows them to discharge this trapped energy.

Other ways this trapped energy can show up is in a nervous tic-like eye blinking, hair pulling, or throat clearing.

Dr. Berceli, in his books like *The Revolutionary Trauma Release Process*, describes how "during any traumatic experience, the body performs this process by contracting the flexor muscles located in the anterior of the body." He's describing the way humans protect ourselves from threat by curling up in a fetal position. We also spend a lot of our time in modernity flexing our front-body muscles: in chairs at work, couches at home, or driving in cars. Anytime you're checking your phone. This causes a lot of imbalanced tension in our flexor muscle groups.

The only time I remember spontaneously tremoring was after a scary car accident. I was the first car through a green light, and a large truck made a right turn on the red light. The truck was so tall that the car behind didn't realize that the light was red and came barreling through. The impact pounded in the front end of my car so badly that it crushed like a can. If it had been a couple of inches closer toward me, I would've lost both of my legs. After detaching myself from the musty-smelling airbag, crawling out the passenger door which hadn't been bent, and sitting on the curb—that's when it happened. My whole body started shivering, as if I was outside exposed on a frozen day. It didn't stop for at least ten minutes, most passersby commented on my intense tremor rather than on the car. Dazed, I didn't think about it then. But once I learned TRE, I recognized what had happened.

The psoas is a large muscle involved in this contraction. The lower insertion, or where this muscle attaches to your body, is on your thigh bones at the top of your upper leg. It's part of the muscle group that flexes our legs. But the bulk of the muscle lies deep inside your body, lining the inside of the pelvis and then running behind the intestine up against your back. If you think of your pelvis as a bowl, from your pubic bone to your hip bones to the spine, the psoas (pronounced *so-ass*) muscle lines the inside of that bowl at the back. Because it's hard to reach, it's challenging to get a satisfactory massage of this muscle, although it holds a ton of tension.

The theory behind other forms of body-based therapy, like Peter Levine's Somatic Experiencing (SE) and Pat Ogden's Sensorimotor Psychotherapy (SP), is that we need to release or complete something trapped in the moment of a trauma. Dr. Levine calls it *sequencing*. In SE practice, it can also look like a tremor.

I studied the first level of SP, and we talked about how there was something that the body still wants to do to recover from a past event. It's like a reenactment of the traumatic episode, except this time the body gets to do what it wanted. Run away, push, kick, twist, or shudder.

In the case of my car accident, the incomplete feeling wants to curl my legs upward to protect them. When I processed a past relationship during SP training, there was a strong desire to push. We used a pillow. In these therapies, allowing the body to finish the movement will release the trauma that's locked into the tissues.

My sense is that this physical release works better for a shocking event, rather than childhood experiences and things that have to do with our relationships. Although, in some of those cases, pushing or kicking while imagining these people can feel great. And attachment trauma may add tension to our muscles through stuck sympathetic activation.

Tremoring is like a completion. It releases the stored energy, but not necessarily in a directed way. The fundamental difference between these other forms of therapy (like SE or SP) and TRE is that tremoring doesn't happen under your conscious control. It's something that the body's innate wisdom knows; it just needs permission.

The psoas muscle, because it's on the inside of your spinal column, runs alongside your dorsal vagus nerve and connects with it into the diaphragm. That's the important nerve that sends messages to your brain. There's an (unproven) theory that TRE can release some of the stored tension in this nerve as well, helping our body rebalance toward our calm nervous system state. If we've been stuck in a low-activation response, these movements can enliven the body and wake up the shut-down nervous system. I find tremoring beneficial in both trauma responses (high and low activation).

I also find TRE helpful after a stressful day or when I can't get to sleep. My body is so accustomed to allowing a tremor that I can perform the technique in my bed, despite its being such a soft surface. With insomnia, I might put my knees in the TRE position, tremor for a few minutes, and then fall asleep easily.

When Dr. Berceli created this activity, he taught a sequence of exercises to tire out our muscles in order for the psoas to shake and release. Now that I've done advanced training with him and his other instructors, I realize that these don't always have to be done. Once your body is used to it, it will tremor when you place your legs in the right position and invite the motion.

While you practice, especially the first couple of times, it's important to notice any negative emotional signals from your body. The two most common reactions are flooding or freezing.

As a refresher, flooding means your high-activation nervous system is feeling overwhelmed. Freezing means your low-activation nervous system is making you feel dissociated. Look for signs of either and move into the stop position if you're in a tremor or don't finish the exercises if you're just getting started.

If any significant physical or emotional pain arises, pay attention to those important signals from the body and stop the practice. I would recommend anyone with physical injuries (or significant trauma or emotional dysregulation) avoid doing this on their own the first few times, as most of it needs to be supported or modified by a trained practitioner.

People with a history of sexual abuse may be uncomfortable with their knees apart (this could be triggering). Some people prefer to be in full control of their body, where release of tension might be overwhelming. Others aren't in tune with their gut instincts and might accidentally push past the Window of Tolerance. In those scenarios, it's best to do it with a guide or at least a support person nearby. I've not seen many people find it distressing, but it certainly can happen.

TENSION-RELEASING EXERCISE

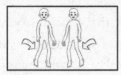

Rolling Feet

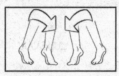

Calf Raises

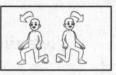

Lunges

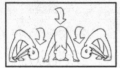

Bending Forward and Turning

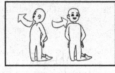

Psoas Stretch

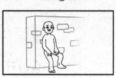

Wall Sit

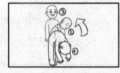

Roll Up Slowly

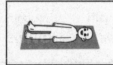

Rest Laying Flat

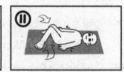

Pause Position: Knees Together

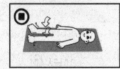

Stop Position: Straighten Legs

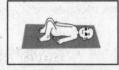

Raise Hips 1-2 Inches

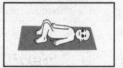

Lower Hips and Rests

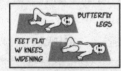

Tremor Position Options

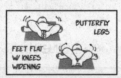

1) Butterfly: Feet Touching
2) Feet Flat on Floor

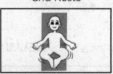

Tremor Starts

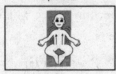

Adjust Position Moving Knees 1 Inch

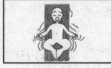

Tremor Moves Up Body

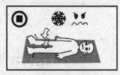

1) Stop if Freeze or Flood
2) Stop after Ten Minutes

Credit: Dr. David Berceli

There's a video of the practice available through the QR code on page xviii.

LET'S PRACTICE—TREMOR

I'll describe the initial exercise sequence that fatigues the surrounding muscles.

In the first exercise, stand with your feet shoulder-width apart and with your knees gently bent. Roll side to side on the soles of your feet. Only go a tiny amount toward the right and left with each breath, not coming right up on the sides of your feet but allowing a small amount of weight there. This grounds you to your body, to establish a connection.

The second exercise is calf raises. For this one, your goal is to try fatiguing the muscle, which doesn't mean pain but just getting tired. They taught us to aim for a 7 out of 10 in fatigue. Basically, I tell my patients that when their brain wants them to stop doing it, that's when the muscle is tired enough. I teach calf raises with the person holding onto a doorknob, wall, or the back of a chair. That way, they don't have to worry about their balance while doing the maneuver. If you're not able to balance on one foot, you can also do this while sitting in a chair and raising a heel. Without any modifications, a calf raise looks like your front foot will raise its heel until most of your weight is on the ball of your foot. That's the big bones just before your toes start. You don't go right up on your toes like a ballet dancer. If a person is an athlete, I cue them to do the exercise slowly because that will tire out the muscle better. To further fatigue the calf, they wouldn't lower all the way to the ground with their heel between every raise.

If you find standing on one foot is a challenge, I recommend doing a kickstand with your back leg, keeping your toes on the ground the entire time. Other people can raise that back foot right up in the air. Again, if you're going to use this option, I would really suggest having something to hang on to for balance.

Do calf raises until you hit that moderate amount of fatigue in your calf muscle. Then, switch and do the same thing with your other leg. If you modify your first leg, I would modify the other one as well—even if only one side has an injury. Then, shake out your leg for a few seconds, the way you would shake some water off your hand.

The next step is a lunge. I recommend continuing to hold on to the object that was helping you balance. With your front foot, keep your knee directly above the ankle during the entire movement, while positioning your back foot a couple of feet behind. As you bend the knee of your front foot into the lunge, your back knee moves toward the floor but shouldn't touch. This means your back foot comes up on the ball of your foot, but keep the weight evenly balanced between both legs. The lunge doesn't involve a single muscle group, and I find some folks feel the fatigue on their back leg before they feel it on their front leg, but for others it's the opposite. A 7 out of 10 in tiredness is a signal to stop doing lunges and switch to the other side. Same as with the calf raises, I rarely recommend doing more than ten lunges. So, for athletes, to tire them out enough, we do them really slowly. Shake out your legs for a few seconds again.

For this next exercise, you widen the stance of your legs beyond your shoulders, as if they're forming a triangle with the floor. Don't go so far that the insides of your thighs are uncomfortable, but that there's a very mild stretch. Keep your knees gently bent, so you don't have stiff, straight legs. Rolling first with your head, and then slowly rolling your spine, you will bend forward with your hands dangling downward. Hold that position for three seconds or one breath. Then, twist your upper body toward one leg, grabbing the foot if that's available to you. Hold there for three seconds or one breath. Twist toward your other foot and do the same. Now, you're going to come back into the middle, but try to see if you can drop a little farther toward the floor.

You can also do this exercise in a chair if doing it standing makes you dizzy or uncomfortable. These exercises all have modifications available, and if you need more than what I'm mentioning, then it's definitely best to try this with a guide the first time or two. Remember to roll up slowly, keeping your knees loose, because lots of people get dizzy if their head travels a large distance too quickly. The heart takes time to catch up to pumping the blood up toward the brain again.

The next exercise is one that I find confusing and past patients don't notice the psoas stretch that it's supposed to create. But I'll describe it here in case it works for you. Standing with your feet hip-width apart, bend your knees again. Put both hands on your lower back where the pockets of jeans would be. From that position, your hands push your pelvic bones or hips about an inch forward. Be very careful not to hyperextend your back; if there's any back pain at all in this position, I would skip the exercise. If it's comfortable for you, you look down over one shoulder toward your elbow, which moves your chin toward that shoulder. Hold it there until you can feel a stretch in the front of your opposite hip. After a couple of seconds, do the same on your other side. Shake out your legs again.

The last exercise is the easiest to describe because it's simple to visualize. For the wall sit, you want a flat surface behind you. Slowly let your feet step about a foot away from the wall. You can go farther out if that's available to you, and you want to drop into an actual sitting position. Most people are just going to bend their knees slightly, because that will be enough. For this position, we recommend holding it for three to five minutes. So, if you find your legs get exhausted, more than a 7 out of 10, move back up the wall and straighten your knees for a couple of seconds. When you feel recovered, drop into the sitting position again, but not as deep. Once you're finished, you bend forward and roll up slowly, keeping your knees loose. Shake out your legs one more time.

Now, move to a yoga mat or carpet, considering whether you want to put a pillow behind your head. I often do, because I've had a whiplash injury (if anyone has had a concussion, I strongly recommend this). Lie flat on the surface and take a few breaths so that your body relaxes from the initial movements.

Check in with your emotions. If they feel heightened, carefully monitor how you respond to the tremor. Or simply try another day.

The first two movements that I teach are the ones that make the tremor stop. Straighten your legs completely with your toes pulling up toward the rest of your body for the *stop* position. Find the *pause* position by bending your knees, moving your feet wider with your soles on the ground, so your knees fall together until they might touch. Holding the pause position makes it easier to restart the tremor if you want to just take a break.

Now that we've practiced how to stop the tremor, let's get it going. The first thing you do is let your feet rest flat on the floor at a comfortable distance, so that your soles plus upper body down to your hips are contacting the mat. Put more weight into the soles of your feet so that you can lift your hips off the mat about one to two inches. Hold this position for about a minute, if that's possible for you. Then, lower your hips back to the floor and spend a minute relaxed.

The tremor itself starts from a position where your feet are flat on the ground, but the inner sides of your feet touch. This makes your knees bend to the right position for tremoring. Another option is the yoga pose called "butterfly," with the soles of your feet touching while the rest of your body lies flat.

Sometimes, the tremor begins quickly in this position, but for many people, they will need to move their knees together or apart to get the movement started. Move your knees symmetrically, both doing the same thing, about an inch at a time.

If the butterfly position (with your knees open) feels too vulnerable for you, definitely do this exercise with a trusted guide to start. Or just stay longer in the wall sit to see if the tremor shows up there, as it often does. I once taught a large group how to tremor using only the wall sit, and almost everybody was successful.

When you do TRE from butterfly or flat feet positions, the tremor often starts as a small shivering movement of your inner thighs, so your knees shake gently. Sometimes, it's bigger, more of a bounce. All of that is normal. Your body knows what it needs.

In my experience, after a few sessions, the tremor often moves upward into the belly and can even travel through the arms or neck. This is the extensors letting go of their tension along the fascia line. While it isn't the psoas muscle directly, it connects to other muscles on the back of the body through fascia or connective tissue.

If a fuller-body tremor happens early, please don't be alarmed. The body knows what it's doing and where it needs to let go of tension.

Dr. Berceli recommends that every session last between ten and fifteen minutes. It's safe to practice daily, but for most people, a maintenance routine is two or three times a week (and he recommends this slower pace when building a practice).

It's really so simple. The body is capable of doing so many wondrous things. I was stunned the first time it happened to me—I didn't know this was possible, and I'm a doctor! Imagine if we taught all children how to release tension in this simple manner. Dr. Berceli did this, in schools and auditoriums around the world.

My dream is that all kids learn how to do these easy physical movements to let go of stress. Imagine how different the world would be if people were carrying around less tension and stuck energy.

Here's a sneak-peek at iffirmations, described in detail later.

What if school children learned to regulate their emotions?
What if work environments had tension-releasing breaks?
What if every person had a body-based toolkit that kept their stress levels low?

What if we believed trauma was something our body naturally handled, so we learn the tools that invite this inner wisdom to work?

SYSTEM SOLUTIONS

CHAPTER 21

Traditions

Now that our body has released some of its tension, we can try the other (cognitive) door to shift trauma responses. We'll start with what humans have always done.

Evolution

When therapists describe traumatic responses, we often go far back into human evolution to explain where they come from. We say that they come from the same place as other mammalian reactions. Mammals are any warm-blooded animal, from whales to dogs to elephants.

A classic example of describing the *high-activation nervous system response* is that of a deer running away from a saber-toothed tiger. These reactions were supposed to be quick movements that would escape danger from a predator, or something natural like a forest fire or river rapids. No mammal evolved to operate from a high-activation nervous system for prolonged periods of time.

The way we describe the *low-activation nervous system response* is the image of a deer that doesn't run or fight—because it didn't work, or they got overwhelmed. Then, the mammal just lies down, hoping that by playing dead, the predator (like a tiger) would give up and go away. This dissociation also helps if the animal does hurt you because you're numb to the experience. The classic animal who does this all the time is the opossum. You may have heard the phrase "playing possum"—pretending to be dead—it's something that this animal does without consciously thinking about it.

217

So do humans.

These nervous system responses have been with us since humans have been around, but they don't always make sense in the modern world. They may not have even made sense ten thousand years ago.

This chapter describes some ways humans preserved knowledge about well-being and mental health, along with some ancient solutions.

Ancient Ways

In most civilizations, they assumed symptoms of mental illness resulted from exposure to a dangerous spirit. This is where things like exorcism, drilling a hole in the skull, and blowing fumes up the lady parts to lure a wandering uterus (the definition of *hysteria*) began.

Ancient Egyptians were among the first to employ the concept of therapeutic recreation. They recommended exposure to music and dancing when people presented with mental illness. They had healing spas with exercise and entertainment. In this time and region, they didn't differentiate between the mind and the body. They believed the cause of low mood was something wrong with the heart or the uterus. Everything in their society was sacred, from architecture to art to relationships. They believed that mental health problems stemmed from a disconnection to what really matters.

I believe this is a fundamental truth, even now.

In many Black African nations, they attribute mental health problems to displeased ancestors or neighbors who have invoked a spirit to attack. A traditional healer is often accessed before a medical doctor. I've visited eight African countries so far, curious to learn how people in rural areas without access to physicians handle such problems. Many clients would take herbal preparations. Some would seek a specialist in spirits, who could chase them out of the home.

Traditional healers do more to explain the meaning behind the condition. They answer questions like why it's happening to the individual and what's causing it—something modern psychology doesn't always offer. When the human brain cares about emotion and story, but modern science insists on checklists and statistics, these concepts don't always translate well.

I remember being in a small hut in Zimbabwe, where a medicine man tossed a dozen small white cowrie shells to the dirt floor. He was predicting my future. I won't get into details, but he turned out to be prophetic about the end of my marriage!

Plants

Herbal preparations have been an ancient formula for mental health across the world. The Celtic women who practiced it were called "white" witches. First Nations people in (what is now called) the Americas have profound relationships with healing plant medicines. One of my patients, an Indigenous Chilean, used to make an appointment at my family practice and describe the herbal medications she tried on her illness. More often than not, she solved her problem before coming. But she felt bad canceling the appointment and so came to tell me about the process. I learned how black cherry extract was helpful for sore joints and gout (it turns out that black cherries have antioxidant properties that lower inflammation).

Charms

Another common belief among various traditions is that of a charm or talisman. Often, the charm is blessed by a spiritual leader or healer. There is significance to a blue eye throughout Egypt, from an allegorical story about a generous deity. Metal amulets have been worn in ancient times throughout the Middle East, often attached to a necklace. For many people who are religious, from historic times until now, their holy book is sacred. Likewise, it was believed that beads or other jewelry with symbols from those spiritual practices would provide safety. In medieval times, astrological symbols were used to invoke protection.

I mentioned volunteering in the Kathmandu Valley of Nepal at a medical school dedicated to serving the rural community. In my time there, I would roll the heavy metal prayer wheels, inscribed with healing phrases (in Tibetan or Sanskrit language). These wheels, and colorful prayer flags, too, send your wishes up into the sky to the spirits.

Bells have special meaning in many Asian and South Asian cultures. I've sat under a humming gong in Myanmar. I've heard the sound of the chimes inviting the monks to take alms (donations) in their saffron robes on the streets of Laos.

In many religions, prayer is an important devotional duty. Interestingly, people who pray or chant have improved mental health and less substance use. While I am not a person who subscribes to a formal religion, I have some spiritual leanings, particularly toward Buddhist philosophy.

If you were raised in a religion that was helpful to you, this can be a powerful antidote after trauma. That being said, rigid and orthodox religions can be a source of trauma as well. If that was the case for you, best to skip this exercise. Sadly, the common interpretation of many religions in modern times has been to invoke shame to control members. It's also a technique in abusive relationships and mimics the same pattern.

Part of the calming feeling in a religious sanctuary is the practice of singing or chanting, which lengthens your exhale and invites the feeling of community.

LET'S PRACTICE—MANTRA

In yoga, one of the mantras is done with finger movements (*kirtan kriya*). I'll describe the movements and then you might try them, along with the ancient or a modern phrase.

Touch the tip of your thumb to the tip of your pointer finger, then move it one by one to your other fingertips, down to your pinkie. That gives you four touch-points if you have all fingers intact and can make these movements. If you can't, using your imagination invokes the same areas of your brain. Move slowly, rhythmically.

In Hindu practice, the phrase said while touching each finger is *Sa* (birth), *Ta* (life), *Na* (death), *Ma* (rebirth). If this speaks to you, or if you were raised in this culture, this might be the phrase to use.

Here are some other suggestions, but I invite you to create one that feels calming and natural:

My journey continues today.
I am safe now.
It will be okay.
Things continue to shift.
Today is brand new.
I am still learning.
May I accept myself.
My healing is possible.
My brain can change.
I accept what is.

Move your thumb to touch each finger for each word in this pattern as a personal mantra.

You might need to change it up from day-to-day, depending on your circumstance and how you're feeling. Always try to keep it hopeful, if not positive.

You might decide to do ten rounds or for one to two minutes. It doesn't have to be a long practice. It's one way to connect ancient traditions with the mind, the body, and the spirit. The full tradition uses mantra (chanting), mudra (hand position), breathwork, and imagery—Indian gurus sure understood the healing power of the body thousands of years ago.

Qigong

Every day, no matter what the weather, my next-door neighbor does *tai chi* (a Chinese martial art) in his backyard. His slow movements and patterns keep him agile.

When I studied *qigong*, I was told that it was the branch of healing of the tai chi practice. The word *chi* or *qi* means "energy." I studied under Master Chunyi Lin in Minnesota, at the Spring Forest Qigong Healing Center.

One of my classmates was studying qigong's impact on chronic pain and finding good results. Another practitioner helps cancer patients in Calgary—Munira Jiwa actually leads the video on the QR linked website. Master Lin says, "Healing comes from alignment of the body, mind, and heart."

The practice is over five thousand years old, but still being done today. It's considered among the Traditional Chinese Medicine techniques. I don't believe humans will do anything for thousands of years if it doesn't have benefits.

The practice requires years to learn all the patterns, so Master Lin distilled the essence into his teachings. I took enough courses that I am considered a "group leader," but by no means do I consider myself an expert.

Slow, gentle movements can remind you of the possibility of safety in your body. The specific movements of qigong restore any blockages in the flow of energy, along *meridian lines* (the pathways that energy naturally takes in the human body). Think of a flowing river. I would recommend qigong for a person who's stuck in a low-activation response, to get them moving easily. It can also help with high activation, because the movements are so slow that it calms the body. As of this writing, the PTSD Association of Canada lists qigong on its website under "Resources," as a coping strategy.

When a person is in dissociation, it's good to practice to return to the body. Let's try it here. While Master Lin keeps his practices close to his chest, he ascribes to wanting the world to have "a healer in every home." I will share a very brief piece of the Spring Forest Qigong experience. Remember, if you have any physical ailments, injuries, or pain issues—it's best to do this with a trained professional.

A video of a led qigong practice is available through the QR code on page xviii.

LET'S PRACTICE—QIGONG

The first part of one's practice is feeling your feet on the ground. If you're standing, or sitting in a chair, place the soles of your feet as flat as you can on the floor. Wiggle your toes and then lay them flat again.

Feel your feet firmly on the floor and imagine a stream of energy connecting the core of the earth flowing up through your body, right through the middle, then up into your head.

Touch your tongue against the roof of your mouth to connect the front and back body. Imagine this energy becomes brighter, and the flow intensifies.

Next, do a gentle bounce to get the rest of your body's energy flowing. You can bounce with softly bent knees, keeping the soles of your feet firmly on the ground. If you're sitting in a chair, allow your core to move up and down as if it was jelly. This isn't a jump—we are not trying to leap. The movement is only about an inch from the knees or from the chair. If it's available to you, keep your wrists loose and allow your arms to dangle overhead and keep bouncing for one more minute. This can be hard on people with sore shoulders; one modification is to keep the elbows bent.

Form your hand into a small cup and pat the top of your head. Then, with the same hand, place it a couple of inches away from your body, just under your belly button. This is the *lower Dantian*, a spot of concentrated energy and healing potential. Allow your imagination to build a ball of bright energy in the lower pelvic area.

Now we will start into a practice that Master Lin calls Joining of the Yin and Yang, to balance the body's energy. Position your hands in a cup shape, about one foot apart from each other. Imagine a ball of energy between your hands, a bright and warm light. Keeping your hands the same distance, as if you were holding a basketball in between, rotate the ball. You can do this from five to thirty minutes, paying attention to your level of fatigue and enjoyment.

To finish, we harvest the energy that was collected in the ball. Rub your hands together until there is some heat in between your palms. Cover your eyes, cupping your hands so you don't press down on them. Then, massage your face, including your ears, and comb your fingers through your hair or across your scalp. If you still have any energy, he recommends forming both hands into a cup and patting your head, across both arms, down your chest and sides, across your stomach and lower back, then down your legs.

Lastly, whether you are standing or sitting, raise your heels so the balls of your feet are the only part contacting the ground. Quickly drop your heels—he recommends doing this five to ten times.

The Vedas

Another ancient way of knowing is Ayurvedic medicine from India. The original Vedic texts are also thousands of years old, and the practice of *yoga* emerged from this as one of many branches of healing.

I trained as an Ayurvedic counselor through the Kerala Academy in California. I don't speak to this very often because I worry about appropriating the traditional practices from a culture that isn't mine. But, again, I don't believe that humans do any practice for this long if it doesn't provide a significant benefit. There's research connecting yoga to healing PTSD, but Ayurvedic medicine encompasses so much more.

In this way of healing, Ayurveda conceives the body hosting three energies, the *doshas*. Every person has a unique balance of these energies, and ill health arrives when there is a shift. Doing an analysis of the energies can help you understand what is out of balance and what can be done to shift back. For example, if you have too much movement energy related to air and space (called *vata*), you'd want to avoid cold foods and irregular routines.

The mental health aspects of Ayurvedic practice line up with the polyvagal theory. Humans would have a dominance of one of the three *gunas* at any time, which directly correlates to each of the trauma responses. *Sattva* is calmness and clarity. This is similar to a ventral vagal state, when the body feels safe and connected. *Rajas* is a restless state, connected to anger and anxiety. Of course, this would correlate to the sympathetic high-activation nervous system response to stress. *Tamas* is stillness, heaviness, and inertia. When there is too much of it, it looks like negligence and depression. This relates to the parasympathetic low-activation, dorsal vagal response to stress. Just as nobody has the same nervous system from minute to minute or day to day, these gunas are also constantly shifting. However, the goal is to spend as much time in a sattvic state as possible.

Imagine that—a modern-day theory that was first described over ten thousand years ago. We have a lot to learn from these ancient practices.

LET'S PRACTICE—BREATH

The word *pranayama* means "breath," which can shift the balance of nervous system responses. While we understand this from physiology, it was also relayed in the Vedic texts.

To shift the mind that is stuck in *rajas*, the high-activation state, choose breath that's slow and focuses on the exhale. My favorite is "bee breathing" or *Bhramari* breath. It's very easy, because it's like a hum. The inhale is slow and luxurious, but the exhale is done by closing your ears with your fingers pressed against its central flap of cartilage, called the tragus, so it blocks your ear canal. You then make a deep hum as you breathe outward, ideally at a low pitch, and for as long as your breath allows. Do this three to five times, experimenting with the tone of the sound.

When this *rajas* energy state is overactive, it's best to create a restful routine, away from crowds. Prevent overwork, stimulating exercise, and even travel. Foods to avoid include those with strong flavors like sour or spicy, but also anything containing caffeine and sugar. The best forms of yoga, if you are keen, would be the ones that are slow moving like *Hatha* or dreamlike, such as *Nidra*. Quiet mindfulness and meditation are useful with a predominance of this *rajas* state.

To shift the mind that is stuck in *tamas*, the low-activation state, the chosen breath is more energetic, like "fire breathing." This is a series of quick exhales with a fast relaxation between, with no active inward breath. You'd use your stomach muscles to push extra air out beyond a normal exhale. Your body naturally pulls air in so that you can continue to take short, fast breaths outward. Because this pattern doesn't allow you to breathe out toxins like carbon dioxide (it's basically hyperventilation), stop if you feel dizzy or if your hands get numb and tingly.

To shift this *tamas* state, move your body every day. Find something new to try, as adventure and interest can reduce *tamas* energy. Avoid heavy foods with meat protein and oils. If yoga interests you, with too much *tamas* state, a fluid practice like *Ashtanga* or a series with flowing poses would be most helpful. If you do meditation, try not to do it in complete stillness, but a guided version with lots of cues to activate the mind.

Here's an Example

Fuyo is renowned for interesting hobbies and explorations. She typically has six projects on the go—from making clay figurines and growing flowers on her balcony, to writing poetry and learning how to swing dance. Her energy level makes her friends tired just thinking about it.

She's been like this since she was small, always curious about everything and trying most of it. She switches jobs every few years. After studying writing in college, she worked as a script supervisor for a disability theater group, then a copy editor for a law firm, inputting artificial intelligence (AI) for web content for arts groups, and now she's freelancing articles about hiking trails in the Pacific Northwest while learning nature photography.

Lately, she struggles to get moving in the morning. On the weekend, Fuyo spent an hour watching a sunlight beam move from the foot of her bed to her legs. Her mind feels as sluggish as her body. Coming up with new ideas seems like a chore. On the days where she forces herself to get outside, she sticks to the same routine—a rooibos latte at the corner coffee shop with a walnut scone dripping in melted butter. Sometimes, she gets it delivered to her apartment. She spends so much time on her couch, its fabric faded on the side closest to the television. She has a heavy feeling from fatty foods and doughnuts that she finds herself craving. Her skin feels greasy, but her skin care routine has been replaced by nightly crying spells.

Fuyo's naturally light *vata* energy has tipped into heavier *kapha*. Just like with the heavy mental *tamas*, she needs to mix up her routine, get moving more, and avoid oily foods.

Indigenous Wisdom

There are many ancient practices among the Indigenous peoples of the world, from the southern hemisphere Aboriginal Australians and Māori in New Zealand, the Guarani in Brazil, and the Quechua of Peru, to the hundreds of First Nations and Inuit tribes scattered in the northern hemisphere across the Americas, Finland, and Russia.

All have profound relationships with their surrounding natural environments, so herbal medicines and land-based practices are an integral part of how they live. In many of these traditions, as has been for centuries, the community is essential to the healing process. Circle dances, steam and sweat lodges, ceremonies marking ritual passages, and prayers to a benevolent Creator are part of many of these cultures. The practices are unique and special. I remember visiting Hokkaidō Island in Japan, where the Ainu people had a magnificent history of carving. We learned of the legend where unusual algae in Lake Akan was considered precious.

Even across Canada, over fifty Indigenous languages are still spoken, despite my government's efforts to eliminate the people and their culture. Traditions like smudging (using the smoke from lit sage, wafting it over one's body to purify), art beadwork, sweat lodges, drumming, and storytelling from elders—these are all profoundly healing practices. Especially for people who survived cultural and social traumas.

In a great tragedy, the Canadian government continues to perpetuate violence against First Nations by failing to enact the Truth and Reconciliation Commission (TRC) recommendations toward collective healing. TRCs have been employed in over forty countries and help move beyond massive problems involving government: including dictatorship in Argentina, geno-cide in Rwanda, civil war in El Salvador, and revolution in Tunisia.

Many of the people who suffered within these larger, systemic traumas continue to have significant related trauma held in their families, communi-ties, and individual body. Healing the collective is essential for all of us.

As you've learned, humans have created ingenious ways of managing stress and tension since the dawn of communication. We explored a few healing practices from traditional life from across the world. This is some-thing our body is innately capable of doing, with many ancient pathways to well-being. It would be ideal if modern medicine didn't forget what the body already knows. While I am so grateful for the technical innovations that I studied as a physician, we must remember there are older, safe, effective (often sacred) practices.

CHAPTER 22

Cultures

I've been privileged to work overseas for most of my career. Before I start this chapter, I'd like to make a mention of *voluntourism*. Working or volunteering abroad can be a damaging and even dangerous practice if not done with a lot of thought. This is when people from the "Global North" journey without knowing cultural norms—they might do harm when they go. It's important to remember that serving abroad typically benefits the traveler more than the country that is visited. Go with curiosity and humility, not a "savior" attitude.

With the organization Global Familymed Foundation that I founded, I've worked in Myanmar and throughout eastern Africa. You've already heard about my time in Nepal.

Through work and traveling, I have been fortunate to visit over eighty countries. I remain conscious of my role as an outside observer and want to preserve my lessons with integrity and respect. So, in this chapter, I'll describe some of the healing practices I've seen on these journeys. These are not always popular traditions nor how all people in a region behave. Please think of them as cultural practices that we can *appreciate* (without *appropriating*, or taking it as if it belongs to us).

Out of the Blue

"Blue Zone" countries are where a large percentage of people live over one hundred years. Researchers study the inhabitants' daily routines to learn why this might happen. One dimension of trauma is that it shortens your life span. Same as anywhere else—stressful events, natural disasters, and developmental trauma happen in these areas. Yet people in Blue Zones live much longer than average. So, what makes a person who lives in a Blue Zone more resilient?

Some concepts from these Blue Zone studies include:

- **Nutrition**

  ❐ A diet full of homegrown vegetables, whole grains, nuts, and legumes—beans, peas, lentils, or chickpeas
  ❐ Meat other than fish once or twice a week
  ❐ In some places studied, people regularly drank moderate (1–2 per day) amounts of red wine, but in other areas, they drank none
  ❐ Many cultures include religious fasting rituals
  ❐ Small portion sizes
  ❐ Coffee in the morning and afternoon

- **Exercise**

  ❐ Practicing tai chi
  ❐ Days full of physical labor on farms
  ❐ Walking up steep slopes of hillside villages
  ❐ Quiet strolls through nature
  ❐ Moving throughout the day, not sitting for most of it

- **Sleep**

  ❐ Between seven to nine hours per night
  ❐ Daytime napping
  ❐ Consistent patterns
  ❐ Quiet times of meditation or mindfulness

- **Socializing**

❑ Having a simple purpose (family, work, or religion)
❑ Multigenerational family household with grandparents looking after young children
❑ A strong social network
❑ Laughter
❑ A pet companion
❑ Family mealtimes

These benefits only exist if you stay in the communities where they occur. Once you move, your habits shift, soon life expectancy and illness trajectories match your destination country.

What are the other superpower ways to keep your body out of the stress responses?

Let's visit some countries with practices that keep the body in a calm, connected, ventral vagal state.

Japan—Imperfections and More

I'd like to introduce you to some ideas from Japan that I haven't seen in the English language.

Wabi-sabi is a concept derived from the Buddhist teaching of impermanence, a sense of accepting that things are always going to change and are rarely perfect.

A common trauma response is that of perfectionism. When a child learns that being good might help them fly under the radar, they might nurture this sense that they must be perfect to be safe. If a person learns to welcome imperfection, they're on the path to healing.

A related term is that of *kintsugi* pottery, which I mentioned at the very beginning of this book. This idea is that if a piece of ceramic breaks, it can be sealed back together with a gold or silver resin. People perceive this art as more beautiful, despite or even because of its cracks and imperfections.

In my mind, this is one of the most extraordinary metaphors relating to post-traumatic growth that I've ever encountered. I keep a piece of kintsugi pottery in a special place in my home to remind me of this concept.

It may seem out of place in a book about trauma, but the concept of *ikigai* is important. Ikigai is the intersection of what the world needs, what brings you joy, and where you can flourish—that is meant to be your purpose.

Finding purpose can motivate you to recover from past trauma, while recovery and helping others on this path can provide purpose to your life. What brings joy during our human experience is *meaning*, whether from work or other activities; and *connection*, which can be with humans, animals, or nature. Because ikigai relates to what the world values and will pay you to do, financial security is also a key aspect of feeling safe.

I've encountered *shinrin-yoku*, or forest bathing, in Japan and in South Korea. Hiking in both countries, I saw more elderly people than I did anybody under the age of sixty. They were always in a group, speaking animatedly with big smiles, wearing bright outdoor gear.

There's been solid research demonstrating the health benefits of spending time in nature. Measurable physical improvements include lowering the neurotransmitters connected to the fight-or-flight stress response, an improved immune system, and better heart function. We can check heart health with heart rate and blood pressure, as well as *heart rate variability*, which refers to beat-to-beat changes. One would assume that consistency is ideal, but it's shifting responses that represent better health. Just like mental flexibility, a change in heart rate determined by the needs of the body shows that you are appropriately adapting to the environment. Lots of people measure heart rate variability through wearable technology.

Research shows that mental health improves when we spend time in nature. Studies show less chronic stress, depression, anxiety, and anger. One Japanese study showed participants gained an extra hour of sleep if they spent time in nature during the day. There's also evidence of changes in brain function through brain imaging and measures of hormone levels.

Some provinces in Canada allow physicians to prescribe a free pass to national parks to patients who can't afford to access these nature preserves. I haven't yet written *"shinrin-yoku"* on the Rx, but I sure am tempted.

These healing lessons are just from a single country. Imagine if we understood the practices of many more of them, how much we would all gain!

LET'S PRACTICE—NATURE

How much time do you currently spend outdoors? Is it an urban environment with lots of cars and shops, or is there anything natural? How close is the nearest park? When's the last time that you touched a tree?

Our body is healthier if we have regular contact with soil; it helps our microbiome (our internal microorganism community). Studies show that our fight against germs, with antibacterial sanitizers for cleaning our hands and countertops, has made us less healthy and resilient. When was the last time you submerged your hands in dirt?

If you have the means and mobility, for the next week, try to contact nature at least once per day. Pay attention to what you experience. Look at the petals of the flower, the veins on a leaf, the rugged bark of a tree. Watch the sunlight dance on ice crystals. Smell the cedar or pine or sticky sap.

How can you bring these sensations into your life at home? Can you nurture any indoor plants? What about a small patio garden with tomatoes? Do you have any pottery made from clay (like terra-cotta)? Do you have any fragrances in your home that invoke the smell of trees or flowers (I don't mean a chemical smell, but a real potpourri or piece of wood)?

Spain—Sleep

Another aspect of healthy living that I learned about in southern Europe and in South America is that of the *siesta*. I've never been good at napping, even when I worked intense night shifts. But sleep is an important part of healing. In cultures where we're consumed with work and achievements, this essential ingredient for a healthy mind and body can get ignored.

I honor the work of the Nap Ministry, who claim "rest is resistance," which is also the title of Tricia Hersey's book. Reclaiming sleep heals generational wounds and the ongoing oppression of overworked racialized bodies.

While there isn't a set amount of time that we should sleep, for an adult, the average set point is seven to nine hours. It doesn't work to get four hours of sleep during the weekday and catch up on the weekends.

There's also a sweet spot with napping. Under ten minutes isn't refreshing, but over thirty minutes throws off your daytime wakefulness and your nighttime ability to sleep. This is all part of your *circadian rhythm*, the internal clock that controls the day-night cycle in humans. All our hormones and neurotransmitters cycle based on the rotation of the earth.

Many people who suffer from PTSD or complex trauma have difficulties with sleep. There's *initial insomnia* when you have trouble getting to sleep after lying down. This is the typical time where the distressed brain dissects the past through the lens of regret and guilt, then worries about the future through the lens of anxiety and dread. The body may feel tense, with amplified pain signals. If you're prone to nightmares, there might be a fear of falling asleep and having to deal with unwelcome memories and disturbing images. Or the bad dreams may disturb sleep with frequent awakening.

South Africa—Community

I've visited the country of South Africa twice and found it magnificent, but also disturbing. The country's recent history is tied up in massive collective trauma. Brutal racism was built into its governance and policies, which remains entangled. With all the progress that Nelson Mandela (who brought temporary peace to the country after imprisonment and reconciliation) and other leaders have achieved, there's still a long way to go. I remember one Xhosa companion telling me that Black communities in the country weren't learning to ride bikes or to swim because these activities connected to trauma and segregation they'd faced.

Yet one of the most healing concepts I've ever learned comes from the same area. *Ubuntu* is a way that people come together with compassion for each other, acting to prioritize the common good. (In fact, most African nations share the concept with a different name.)

Throughout the COVID-19 pandemic, and when I think about the climate crisis, I wish this idea would catch on like a virus. Countries where individualism and the bootstrap mentality (the fallacy of "pulling up by one's bootstraps" despite social obstacles) dominates is a signal that we don't look after each other. But when it comes to trauma, there's nothing more important.

Collectivist cultures have less mental health ailments. Individualistic ones, where every human is "out for themselves" and can't rely on community care, struggle much more. In many ways, hyperindividualism is a cultural trauma response. When people learn that others don't look after them, they behave in ways to reinforce becoming self-secure. It starts as a *scarcity mind-set*, that there's not enough for everyone. Too much focus on individual ego and gain creates inequity, the largest systemic source of trauma.

When a person shifts their mental framework toward the belief that people can't be trusted, healing comes through small gestures of caring. Unfortunately, once the brain has been traumatized, we're more likely to pay attention to the opposite—when people fulfill your expectations and act in ways that are mean, violent, or self-serving.

Some nations have fallen into cyclical patterns of violence and greed, initially to survive, but then becoming ingrained into culture. Moral compassion isn't taught to the next generation, only the survival skills.

HERE'S AN EXAMPLE

For most of her childhood, Faith believed people were out to get her. This made sense, considering all that she'd been through. It wasn't until she landed at her aunt's house that she saw that kind people exist. She'd watch Aunt Doris cook up a batch of chili and put it in plastic cups that she would then give to people sitting at the steps of the homeless shelter on the next block. Her aunt was involved in community organizing, often helping with fund-raising efforts for sports centers to give young people a place to be safe and have fun.

Playing basketball was something Faith had always loved to do, no matter what school or city she found herself in. She never let herself get close to any of her teammates, knowing she would probably move on. But Aunt Doris would show up to all of her games, inviting the team back to their small apartment for chips and seven-layer dip. Faith eventually realized that she could count on those girls; they had her back. Growing up, this wasn't something she could've ever imagined.

One evening, Faith was at one of her teammates' homes doing homework. While her friend wasn't looking, the girl's brother groped Faith. In the past, she wouldn't have bothered to tell anybody, but in this new home, she trusted the community and thought they'd believe her. When she told her aunt what happened, it was the first time that somebody had ever seemed to care when she was hurt.

Together, they made a plan to make sure that Faith wouldn't be in that kind of dangerous situation again. They asked her friend if any of her sisters were being harmed in the home. Sadly, her friend admitted this brother had inappropriately touched one of her sisters. Aunt Doris helped her friend navigate a conversation with their mother, so that the family could figure out together what to do. While Faith wished this kind of support had been there for her when she was a child, it was a turning point in her life to see that her aunt cared for her in this way. And that families could turn difficult things around.

Cuba—Group Work

In all the times that I have worked overseas, by far the greatest number of physicians deployed to work in another country to help an underresourced area came from Cuba. I saw Cuban cardiologists and pediatricians working in rural Laos. The Cuban system of socialism means that the doctor and the janitor at the hospital get paid the same amount, but there's obviously a lot more training and probably reverence for the physician. I will not pretend that it's easy (one of my colleagues at the refugee clinic escaped the regime)—every country has nuances, but I certainly saw a lot of good done through these Cuban physicians.

In Cuba, medical care is known for integrating the mind and the body instead of seeing them as separate. Every person can access a psychologist if they wish. As it's integrated into the health system, there's less stigma and more access. Family and community are integral to Cuban society, so group interventions are acceptable. Group medical visits help a person who has been through trauma feel validated and heard. They can learn about healing practices through other group members, being a witness and support on one another's journeys.

If you're interested in finding a group therapy session, there are many offered through organizations like the YMCA/YWCA, women's centers, and immigrant support groups. Some might build on cultural practices. Others might follow a formula like DBT, which is generally explored as group therapy. Solid research backs groups for addiction; there's support in such programs and learning environments.

LET'S PRACTICE—GROUPS

Are there any groups available to you? I searched the website Psychology Today and found trauma-specific groups across the United States and Canada. There are also groups for mothers suffering from postpartum depression, group anger-management skills, groups for grieving the loss of a family member, for transgender folks navigating social issues, and many more.

Many arts and creative therapies, including performance, are in a group setting and are often a fun and playful way to address trauma. Something to be cautious of in this setting is *vicarious trauma*, suffering from hearing about others' problems and pain.

In this chapter, we explored only a few concepts that I was exposed to while journeying through other countries. Each culture has unique healing practices. There is no single way to live, to heal, to connect, or to grow.

Part of being *culturally humble* is the realization that each society has its powerful practices and is innately resilient.

Rather than wishing we would all assimilate to become one model of success, we would be better off recognizing that we learn and prosper through our differences and ways of being. I've been privileged to explore other cultures, many of which are not so traumatized as the one where I live. With greater adoption of ideas like healing from nature, connecting to the body's intrinsic healing properties, and community care—we'd have a healthier world for all.

CHAPTER 23

Routine

The goal of this chapter is to develop a lifestyle aimed at healing traumatic responses in the brain and body. Humans have undergone shock (event) and attachment (relational) trauma for centuries, and we have evolved many ways of maintaining the best health possible under these circumstances.

Let's go through a typical day of a person who works nine to five on their job site, thinking about our choices in the context of trauma.

I will not describe all the research, because I promised you a book that wasn't very academic—but you can find that in the resource section of the website (through the QR code on page xviii), if you're interested. Remember that scientific research is always changing, and so I'm presenting the most current information. But science is under constant investigation, and recommendations change the more we understand. An important disclaimer is that you might need a medical opinion about some of these suggestions, so ask your health-care team to collaborate on your personal routine.

7 A.M.

The first thing that many of us do in the morning is take a shower. The question here is—hot or cold? While my preference is heat, there's evidence to suggest that exposing yourself to cold or cycling between the two temperatures is best for your system.

According to Wim Hof (the Dutch "Iceman" who jumps into cold water and does an adaptation of ancient breathing exercises), cold temperatures can help regulate the nervous system and produce *endorphins*, the hormones responsible for feeling happy. Certainly, if your body is stuck in a lower activation response, the cold would wake it up. But this technique works not by irritating the system but by enhancing it. Your body adapts to cold temperatures. Research shows it can improve sleep, reduce stress, help with concentration, and increase energy levels. It can also cause harm to a body, so approach this with caution outside of your personal shower.

8 A.M.

A warning to this tip—it has to do with food. It's worth reflecting on your relationship with eating and weight before deciding if this is safe to try. This is not diet advice, but energy advice and the key is noticing if the practice (should you decide to try) gives you more or less energy.

Do we eat breakfast, or do we skip it to practice *intermittent fasting*? This is when a person limits the hours during the day that they eat to a maximum of eight or ten hours, rather than grazing throughout the day. This practice can change brain neurotransmitter levels.

The guidelines suggest skipping one of your meals. If you're going to choose a ten-hour window, and you want to eat dinner around six p.m., you would eat your breakfast midmorning. Alternatively, you could start your day with a hearty meal and then wind down your intake by five to six p.m.

Be extremely careful incorporating this method if you've ever had issues with food. Anyone with an eating disorder should consider intermittent fasting carefully because it could cascade into other unhealthy eating behaviors. Diabetics generally can't use this method of eating. If you have tried it, what do you notice about your own mood and energy level? Early evidence is mixed, so it might benefit some but not all.

9 A.M.

I'm going to use the example of road rage to illustrate how your nervous system is in charge of so many minor tasks throughout your day. If you're the kind of person who's constantly shouting at passing cars, grinding your teeth, and white-knuckling your steering wheel, this could reflect too much of the "fight" energy from the sympathetic nervous system.

When you notice road rage, it's a great opportunity to shift your nervous system—in the moment. When you notice it's overactive, there are many small things you can do to calm it down. Most of these are techniques to draw attention away from your stress. Try to distract your brain by noticing five colors in the passing cars, ten license plates with vowels, or naming the manufacturer of cars you see on the road. Look for people walking their dogs, or drinking from a cup, or wearing sneakers. Turn on the radio or play music from your device that's more calming. Helping your mind pay attention to more neutral things is a superb skill to practice.

10 A.M.

Take that coffee or tea break. When your activated nervous system kicks in from the stress of the workday, a straightforward way to rebalance is to counteract with digestion. Swallowing or going to the bathroom is enough. If you engage anything along the gastrointestinal tract, that will activate the parasympathetic, low-activation "rest and digest" system. So, keep a water bottle handy and sip from it often, to prevent getting overloaded from stress. And don't ignore the body cues to visit the washroom. It's a fantastic way to practice *interoception*, or listening to the signals from our body—something we've learned to ignore when we've been in situations where we had to suppress those internal messages.

When you're thinking about tea, consider an herbal preparation that can actively work on the mind. Nervines are herbs that relax the body. This includes skullcap, passionflower, catnip, valerian, and chamomile. Note that they can make some people very sleepy rather than just calm, so that might be more of a bedtime routine if this is the case for you. This summer, I started growing wild chamomile in my new herbal medicine garden, so I'll make homegrown tea soon!

Latifa Pelletier-Ahmed, a Canadian herbalist, runs a group "medicine walk" in both the city and the countryside. When she studied in the United

Kingdom, she observed that they didn't mention anxiety or depression to the students. Instead they described herbs as an effective way to nourish the nervous system. Other helpful herbs include *Ginkgo biloba*, which improves brain function. Bitters stimulate digestion and calm the nervous system. Notably, Latifa recommends we seek Indigenous knowledge in our areas. There are always ethical concerns with herbs and essential oils in terms of how they are sourced and impact endangered species. Every region will have different wild varieties, so a local expert familiar with native species is ideal.

II A.M.

Incorporate some rhythmic movement into your day. Whether it's tapping each foot one at a time on the floor or tapping your palm against your thigh. You could even tap on your collarbone points and bring some EFT into your workday. Drumming with your fingers on the desk works if you're not in an open-concept office. Patterned and repetitive movement includes taking a walk, so make an excuse to refill your water or go check in on a colleague.

Many brains benefit from the Pomodoro Technique, where you concentrate on learning or working for a set amount of time and then take a break. There are apps and websites that can guide this, typically doing the activity for twenty-five minutes and then taking a five-minute break.

So, adding these two things together might mean that you take a break to do something rhythmic. Dance break in the kitchen, anyone? After a few sessions, a longer break is recommended—perhaps once an hour, refilling that water bottle.

NOON

We're going to enjoy a lunch prescribed by a psychiatrist and nutritionist at Harvard. Dr. Uma Naidoo, in her book *This Is Your Brain on Food*, describes the nutrition you need to consume when you've been diagnosed with different psychiatric conditions. Like me, she's uncertain that the symptom complexes in the DSM reflect a distinct illness, but she agrees that the environment affects neurotransmitters and hormones.

While this is her advice, food preferences are often cultural and the eating experience is often social, so there are no absolutes. As with the earlier warning, if disordered eating is part of your coping strategies, this may not be the best suggestion for you.

If we're at work, let's presume that the sympathetic nervous system is the one in overdrive, as you are moving and in a potentially stressful environment. So, for lunch, we are going to have a diet tied to reducing anxiety in the brain. Fried food, sweetened drinks, or heavy red meat leads to anxiety and unhealthy changes in the gut bacteria. Not only do high-fat foods correlate with anxiety in research trials, but eating these will cause the part of the brain related to PTSD (the hippocampus) to shrink more than it already does from trauma alone. Sugar and easily digested carbohydrates, like white rice or potatoes, are also suboptimal to a brain that has been through trauma.

Likewise, keeping energy drinks and caffeine in moderation is a good idea. Certain coffee shops deliberately put in four or five times the amount of caffeine in a single drink. It's easy to build up a tolerance without noticing. Dr. Naidoo recommends a maximum of 400 mg per day, before midafternoon.

We've talked about what to avoid; but what's the best food to eat to lessen the symptoms of anxiety and the sympathetic nervous system? According to Dr. Naidoo, dietary fiber is the principal ingredient that promotes growth of healthy bacteria in the gut. Things like beans, brown or black rice, bran, fruits with skin, oats, and almonds or walnuts. Another nutrient that's helpful in reducing anxiety through anti-inflammatory properties in the brain is *omega-3 acid*. Fish and other seafood are the best source, and switching your cooking oil to avocado or olive oil is healthier. Vegetarian sources of omega-3 acids include flax or chia seeds, tofu, and the sea algae that fish eat. Fermented foods—kimchi or sauerkraut, miso or tempeh, cider vinegar, and plain yogurt—also improve the microbiome and decrease anxiety.

I was speaking at a conference in South Korea a few years ago, where I visited a clinic whose physician prescribed different kinds of kimchi (salted, fermented vegetables) to help with his patients' anxiety. He even did a stool analysis in his office to check the patients' results!

Lastly, tryptophan is an ingredient needed to form the "feel-good" neurotransmitter (brain signal) serotonin and can be obtained through dietary sources like chickpeas (including hummus) or turkey. A cup of chamomile tea or a turmeric latte, with a handful of blueberries for antioxidant properties (which cleans up damaging molecules like Pac-Man), is a great way to finish our calming lunch break.

1 P.M.

Is there any way to spend some time on your own? The brain that survived trauma needs both time for connection and time for solitude.

If your work environment promotes one of these scenarios, is there a way to find yourself more of the other? Schedule a team meeting if you've been working alone. Wander into a solo room if you are in an open-space cubicle arrangement.

Just as the work of healing from trauma includes learning to feel safe both alone and with others, we can practice this in micro-moments during the day.

2 P.M.

Have you remembered to move your body? In her book *The Extended Mind*, science writer Annie Murphy Paul describes how movement and gestures can stimulate the brain. In fact, our memory works better when we are in motion. You get extra benefit by being somewhere that inspires creativity: an interesting space or getting into nature. Anytime the brain is functioning better, it means that rewiring toward safety is more available to us.

3 P.M.

Time for a healthy snack—to keep our digestive tract working and our calm nervous system on board. Let's think about the microbiome, all the bacteria that live in the gut, and get their needs met too. Grab a kombucha or kefir—these fizzy, fermented drinks replenish the good bacteria in our system. One of my colleagues, the department head of psychiatry at the University of Calgary, conducts research on pills full of good microbiome (fecal transplant pills made in the lab) to improve your mental health. Dr. Valerie Taylor has studied different conditions through the microbiome lab. Even encapsulated, uninformed people think it sounds gross, but it's truly exciting research. Imagine how revolutionary it will be when we all understand that changing the bacteria that live in your body improves your state of mind.

4 P.M.

As you drive home, find ways to relax the body and make a clear transition from the workday. Listen to music—perhaps sing or hum along. It's not just fun, it's also scientifically proven to rebalance the nervous system. And, by ignoring any shame signals telling us we aren't good enough at singing, it might mean we get better at ignoring the shame signal at other times.

Podcasts are another significant source of information and entertainment. I love plugging into educational ones, but the key is attending to how your nervous system feels when you're listening. When I meet patients for the first time at the addiction clinic, I often share a list of recommended episodes including Stephen Porges on *Bulletproof Radio* and Bessel van der Kolk being interviewed on *On Being*. Any episodes with Bayo Akomolafe or Resmaa Menakem are worth finding. Brené Brown, a researcher known for her studies of shame and vulnerability, has also started podcasting; her friendly voice always brings a smile to my face. These suggestions are heavily weighted toward mental health professionals, but maybe you want to listen to something more funny or entertaining? Remember adrienne maree brown and her sister's apocalyptic podcast? The key is noticing what makes your nervous system feel restored.

5 P.M.

Meditation can be a hard task when a person's brain is programmed to send danger signals. When you quiet your mind, these signals can sound even louder. Mindful practices, simple acts like driving or walking, can be just as powerful. When you're in motion, on your way home perhaps, what can you notice about where you are? How many clouds are in the sky? What do the trees look like, and are they moving in the wind? Be careful not to be too distracted if you're driving, of course.

You will feel a sense of awe when you notice more details about your surroundings. The sparkle of sunshine reflecting off ice. The sound of a river bubbling. The joy of a dog running with a stick in its mouth. Noticing how some people dress for one season while others seem prepared for a completely different one. Things that you notice that are beautiful or playful are best for the nervous system. You can also practice mindful eating or mindful presence. It's all about being more aware or attuned to the moment.

6 P.M.

For dinner, our body may feel more relaxed after a busy workday (unless home is more chaotic), and we don't want to allow it to tip into the underactive nervous system response. Let's consult Dr. Naidoo's book again, this time regarding the symptoms of depression. Here she mentions probiotics (which grow our healthy gut bacteria), often found in plain yogurt but also tempeh, miso, and the other fermented foods we considered for lunch. Cheeses like Cheddar, mozzarella, or Gouda also have active probiotic cultures. She mentions prebiotics as well (which supports the process), including beans and other legumes, bananas, garlic, onions and leeks, or asparagus. Her recommendation for a lower activity nervous system is the Mediterranean diet, which is mostly plant-based and does not involve anything processed—so avoid food that's factory-made with many ingredients. Ultimately, this may not be suitable to your ethnic background, so whatever is culturally appropriate or easily sourced locally is best—the goal is selecting whole foods rather than packaged.

Dr. Naidoo recommends avoiding any artificial sweeteners. The best source of omega-3 fatty acids, that component of our brain cells, comes from fish like salmon, mackerel, tuna, herring, or sardines. Edamame, wal-nuts, and chia seeds are good plant-based sources. Having many colors of vegetables on the plate is good for vitamins and minerals. Sometimes iron deficiency is linked to depression, so rotating shellfish with lean red meat, or snacking on pumpkin seeds is a good way to replenish iron levels. I eat more vegetarian food, so pop an "iron fish" into soup or stew pots!

How we eat is just as important as what we eat. Sometimes, it feels good to be alone and read a book. Being away from a work environment, so you get an actual break, is great for staying in our calm nervous system (which digests). Being in the company of others—whether pets or people—might also help you stay in that regulated and connected state.

7 P.M.

We've previously discussed the role of herbal medications, so I'd like to focus here on micronutrients. These fuel the activity within our body. This includes making the chemicals that send messages between brain neurons and throughout the body using neurotransmitters and hormones. Some experts recommend taking B-complex vitamins, vitamin D, zinc, and mag-nesium. More research is coming out about how many of us are deficient in these essential substances. It makes little sense to me that a trauma response comes from a lack of nutritional building blocks, but it certainly would help to have them all available while rewiring the brain. Eating your vitamins with food is important because many of them need fat to be absorbed.

8 P.M.

Connecting with others is an important way to practice your attuned ner-vous system, what we called ventral vagal. This could be spending time with your partner or kids, giving a parent or friend a phone call, teaching your pet a new trick, or just connecting deeply with yourself through medi-tation or prayer. Connection is a deeply important practice for humans; too many of us are isolated. If you're in a small space, nurturing a fish or a lizard can be a source of joy, meaning, and connection.

9 P.M.

Turn off your devices to prepare for the best sleep possible. Reading and listening to music are good alternatives. An electronic screen with blue light tells your body that it's daytime and doesn't allow it to produce its natural hormones that will regulate your circadian rhythm, the internal clock inside your brain and body. Normally, the hormone *melatonin* would increase around this time to help you get tired. Blue light confuses the body enough that this hormone doesn't show up.

Consider any of the body-based calming practices from the previous chapters at this time, including Havening or TRE tremoring. Having healthy habits that involve journaling, self-compassion meditations, and a gentle self-care routine is often beneficial. But you're the expert on your body, so it's important to pay attention to how much energy (spoons) you have left and what feels best in your nervous system.

10 P.M.

For ideal sleep, having a quiet brain is the best. Actively turn off all the worries and regrets with an app with "colored" noise or a gentle guided meditation. There are lots of free ones, including on YouTube, but using a fan or humidifier works if you don't have access to low-cost internet. If you have difficulty falling asleep, and you have a set of earbuds or headphones that differentiate right from left ears, binaural beats for insomnia are free online. It's filtered music that sends different signals into each half of your brain; people find it useful for better sleep or for lowering stress.

Many people do nightly prayers as part of a spiritual practice. This is another thing that will calm the body, a routine that encourages health and connects them to their community.

11 P.M.

Keep the same routine during the weekday and weekends. Our system runs on an internal clock of hormones and neurotransmitters, which is hard to switch for a couple of days every week. Shift work and jet lag are hard on those chemicals. Whenever I had to deal with that, I would anticipate by shifting my clock slowly toward the place where I was going.

Your body's immune system works the hardest when you sleep. It's also when you reconsolidate (form storage of) memories from the day.

Bad dreams are more likely when there's unresolved trauma from the past trying to figure out its meaning in the present. The more habits you practice calming your nervous system, the more you process the past so it doesn't sneak into the present, the better you will sleep.

Putting a lotion or oil on your hands and feet, one with a soothing smell, is a small act of self-care. It's one of the Ayurvedic techniques I studied.

There are so many options for a night routine, like:

- Drink warm tea, milk, or alternative mylk
- Pet an animal or get cozy in a soft blanket
- Essential oil diffusers
- A fan or other white noise, even a small water feature
- A cool-mist humidifier is nice on the skin
- A gratitude journal
- Reading a book in the bath
- A facial hydrating mask

Good night, sweetheart.

You are loved.

CHAPTER 24

Self-Talk

Every human has a voice inside their head. Sometimes, it rattles off a list of what we need to pick up at the grocery store. Other times, it tells us all the lousy things we've ever heard about ourselves or overanalyzes the conversation we've had. This is called negative self-talk or the *inner critic*.

When a person has been through trauma, the voice gets preoccupied and loud.

It scans the environment for danger:

Who is that guy? I don't remember seeing him in the neighborhood before.
I better put my bike inside in case he wants to steal it.

It might scan the environment inside your body:

What's going on with that twitch in my eyelid? Am I having a stroke?

Creating new patterns for this inner voice is a substantial part of therapy and a major focus of the top-down approach. In traditional talk therapy, there's attention to what you're thinking and why, learning new ways of thinking, and coaching yourself to make changes.

Here's the alphabet soup of therapy names—don't worry about remembering them. Talking about your thoughts is the basis of cognitive behavioral therapy (CBT); also its cousins cognitive processing therapy (CPT) and acceptance and commitment therapy (ACT), as well as a large part of dialectical behavior therapy (DBT). With Internal Family Systems (IFS), the voices are even more important, as they're seen as distinct characters. I'll go over my favorite aspects of each of these briefly, then share my absolute favorite self-talk tools—imagery and iffirmations.

Talk Therapy Targets Thoughts

I studied in medical school that CBT is the gold standard (the best) for trauma and pretty much every other mental health diagnosis. It has the most rigorous studies and the largest number of them. Its target is discovering when the voice inside your head is misleading.

The basis of CBT is finding unhelpful thoughts and changing them, because the thoughts lead to behaviors. You act on what your brain tells you to do. Cognitive...behavioral, see?

Techniques used in CBT might be ideas you're already familiar with. We've discussed pros and cons. Everyone rates their choices to decide which to pursue.

Another tool I really like is to "look for exceptions." Imagine that your brain, because it's been through trauma, expects bad things to happen. If you notice when this hasn't been true, that plants a seed of doubt in the pattern of hopelessness. One that can be nurtured in therapy. *When did things go well for you? When did you have success?*

In CBT models, there's an assumption that your brain is online. That the choices you make involve the thinking brain (neocortex). But in trauma, that's often not true. A lot of actions are reflexes, coming straight from your "alarm center."

So, if a therapist asks you to write the ABCs and they're talking about antecedents, behaviors, and consequences—that might seem like too much to do when the brain just wants you to run away. Not only that, but your brain isn't thinking about those ABCs. It just wants to avoid the threat, no matter what.

My other hesitation about using too much CBT is that it can feel shameful. If you're told your brain is full of unhelpful thoughts and you already tell yourself that there's something wrong with you, this therapy might confirm the belief. Remember, your brain is sending these messages to protect you.

We should be grateful to that inner critic, maybe call it an "inner protector" instead. It's rational to be anxious after trauma.

Modified for Trauma

When a person encounters trauma, CBT morphed into CPT to examine the "unhelpful beliefs" specific to the traumatic episode. Therapist and client walk through the event and see which thoughts are stuck. It's set up to take a dozen sessions, with lots of homework. In complex trauma, it would take much longer to go through it all.

As we've mentioned before, you can't experience trauma in a calm body. So, this exposure-style therapy has a lot of potential if you can stay calm while you do it. You need an accessible thinking brain, though, which isn't always the case when danger alarms are ringing. And, when the danger was very real, it can feel like gaslighting to tell yourself new messages.

Values-Based

A more recent spin-off practice from CBT is ACT. I'm a fan of this approach because it is more individualized and recognizes that each person has their own priorities and goals.

ACT still takes a lot of brain power. Just like DBT, there are a lot of acronyms and steps. When your thinking brain isn't fully available because it's locked in a trauma response, this can be too much to remember.

There are interesting aspects to ACT. Think about the name—*acceptance* and *commitment*. Learning to accept that trauma has happened and committing to improving your life, anyway. That's a powerful idea.

Unlike DBT that has four branches, ACT has six facets. It also has some unusual language—like "unhooking from fused" ideas, "experiential avoidance," and "examining your Self as Context." In a brain that's still got alarms going off loudly, these words could further clutter the mind.

When you look at what ACT teaches, though, it can be helpful. Here are some of the main takeaways that I got from taking Dr. Russ Harris's foundations course and the one focused on trauma:

- No emotions are bad. Just let them flow through, as they're constantly changing.
- You can change foundational beliefs. This starts by noticing them and asking if they are true or if they served a purpose that's no longer helpful.
- Focus on what matters to create the most meaningful changes.

From C to D

The reason DBT is called *dialectical* is the concept of "dual," that there are two aspects to the therapy: change and accept.

The "accept" branch of DBT means you learn to live with certain situations and remain grounded in the present. They use the tool of mindfulness, which comes from many other ancient traditions. With DBT, mindfulness is learning to accept the reality in front of us and to be attuned to the truth of our surroundings. The other "accept" branch has to do with distress tolerance—how to get through something painful that's unavoidable.

An excellent aspect of the distress tools is that the creator of DBT, Dr. Marsha Linehan, suggests body-based practices. She recognized that when your brain is upset or agitated, you can't always think your way out of the problem. So, she includes things like the cold reflex, where you stick your hands in ice water or splash it on your face to shift your nervous system into "rest and digest" mode. She talks about doing activities you enjoy to distract from your problems. Or activities that are hard to ignore—strong tastes or smells—to shift your focus.

LET'S PRACTICE—DE-STRESS KIT

I often suggest that patients create a small toolkit for distress tolerance. Put things in a bag that you grab along with your wallet and phone:

- A stone for grounding and to feel its texture
- A scent like an essential oil or a hard mint
- A jawbreaker or Pop Rocks candy to enliven your mouth
- A fidget spinner or ring

What are the objects that you could put in a distress kit? (Let's call it a de-stress kit.)

Think about the senses:

What could you look at? What could you taste? What could you feel? Think back to ASMR. *What could you smell? What could you listen to?*

If a kit isn't available, there's always something in the environment. You may have heard of the 54321 technique, whereby you look for five things to see, four to feel, three to hear, two to smell, and one to taste. For many patients, this causes frustration, as there isn't always this much variety around.

Instead, if you don't have a kit on you, look for three things in the space that are beautiful or unusual. Allow your mind to focus on what's different about it. This could be a color, the shape of a lamp, or a carpet. It could be a puffy cloud with two colors and shaped like a mouse.

Next, find three textures—the furniture or some wood, the floor or grass. If possible, touch each of them and notice how they feel. Soft or hard? Smooth or bumpy?

The more you notice in your surroundings, and the more senses you use, the more present you will feel in the moment. That way, your brain can't wander to the painful past or fearful future.

The "change" branches of DBT are emotional regulation and interpersonal effectiveness. These skills help shift your emotional responses to achieve more of what you prefer.

Like any successful therapy, the first steps to this branch are noticing. *What emotions are happening in your mind? What sensations in your body?* Some people who've learned to dissociate as a protection mechanism don't recognize nuanced emotions. They may start by just labeling them comfortable or uncomfortable.

The primary tool Dr. Linehan mentions to move toward a new emotion is that of opposite action, where you act on the exact opposite of what is showing up in the body. *If you're feeling shame, what are you comfortable sharing with someone safe? If you're noticing anger, what can you do that is kind or serves another person's needs?* To be honest, I haven't had a lot of success with this technique. Once you've been through trauma, reflex emotions and actions are hard to "talk ourselves out of," and sometimes they're the safest option.

The effectiveness aspects of DBT is where I get lost in the weeds. There are many acronyms (FAST, GIVE, DEAR MAN) that are hard to remember. Harder in a brain where the neocortex is offline. One aspect that this piece shares with ACT is a focus on values, which are always important.

> Who do you choose to be? What matters to you?

Therapists often deliver DBT in a group setting and with homework assignments to practice. Groups aren't serene environments for all people, especially those who attune to the emotions of others (empaths). If your thinking brain isn't always firing, with repeated exposure to the ideas, many will sink in. They'll become a part of your routine or new reflexes. This has been the case for some of my patients; others felt it was gaslighting.

It's puzzling that they typically offer DBT only to people diagnosed with borderline personality disorder. If it were up to me, we'd teach mindfulness, distress tolerance, emotional regulation, and interpersonal effectiveness to schoolchildren. Every human needs these tools. But, for me, I'd teach the body as the doorway into these new patterns.

DBT uses a tool that I frequently incorporate into my sessions: imagery.

Guided Imagery

It's easy to guess what imagery is like.

Imagine you're on a beach. Smell the sea and taste the salt air.

There are phone apps and YouTube videos with imagery exercises. But there's a way to take it up a notch for the brain that's experienced trauma. By helping a person restore calm to the body, imagery takes you to a peaceful place. But to get the brain participating, instead of leaping to the reflex of fight-or-flight or paying attention to the internal alarm bells, an extra helpful feature is distraction.

When participating in an imagery exercise, then it's called interactive. When I do it in sessions with my patients, it's Interactive Guided Imagery because I give them cues about how to best distract at every stage of the imagery. I studied this through the Academy for Guided Imagery.

Think of imagery like a dream—one where you have control, so you can keep it safe, and one where you want to invoke the most pleasant sensations (physical feelings, emotions, and hopes). A recording of a longer version of this exercise is available through the QR code at page xviii.

LET'S PRACTICE—THE BEACH

Imagine you're on the beach. Are you wearing flip-flops or are you barefoot? How close do you want to get to the waves? If you go into the waves—imagine lovely, soothing, warm water caressing your feet. Look behind you and count your footprints. Imagine they fade as the water passes over them, softening into sand.

Count six steps out loud. Notice the smell and taste of salt in the sea air. How hot is the sun? Would you want to be wearing a sunhat or sunglasses? Can you smell coconut sunscreen?

Picture the sun right on the horizon. What three colors do you see in the sky? The sky glows and the air is still warm. You can hear birds chirping behind you—are they tropical? Can you see their colors?

You notice one fly upward, drifting with long wings. Its silhouette glides against the setting sun and colored clouds. It looks so beautiful. There's a soft smile on your salty lips.

Internal Family

We've been talking about the singular voice in our head. But what if we unlock many voices? I don't mean "multiple personality"—what we now call dissociative identity disorder (outside the scope of this book).

Dr. Dick Schwartz noticed that many of his patients would talk about parts of their mind stuck at the ages and beliefs when trauma happened. He called these the Exiles. Then he noticed other parts were protective. He named these Firefighters and Managers. This makes sense from the polyvagal theory and what we've already learned about the brain. Firefighters want to run away or fight the fire. Managers disconnect from the emotion and just handle the problem.

In his therapy, called Internal Family Systems (IFS), these parts live inside all of us. Sometimes the Exiles take over, with thoughts and actions coming from a childlike part trying to cope while under threat. By thinking of them as stuck younger parts of ourselves, we can approach them with more compassion.

In IFS, we learn to spend more time as the Integrated Self, while being able to have internal conversations with all these other parts. The voice inside your head turns into a crowd.

From a trauma perspective, I love the possibility of having the adult Self soothe the younger parts that are still in pain. It's a great way to reparent.

The self-talk encouraged in IFS is one of clarity, speaking to each of the parts whether they're an Exile or a protector, and getting curious about what they believe. There are eight C's that Dr. Schwartz talks about in the concept of Self, but again—the traumatized brain doesn't like to remember long lists, so don't focus too much on these. These C-words that signal you're operating from Self are curiosity, compassion, clarity, connectedness, creativity, courage, confidence, and calm.

The most beautiful part about IFS is compassion—that our integrated Self can offer it to these parts that feel shame, self-loathing, guilt, fear, or worse. Then we can figure out where these thoughts and feelings came from, so the Self helps them to heal.

Because each person will have different parts stuck at different ages and stages, this therapy is often done with a trained professional.

Iffirmations

Iffirmations are one of my favorite tools to help people create new possibilities. If you follow me on TikTok, this may have been the first video you saw (it got over a million views).

You've probably heard of affirmations. It's when you say a phrase in your mind, like a repeating mantra, that you want to be true. You may believe it, you may not. But your goal is to repeat the phrase until it becomes reality.

Think, "I am a star. I am a star." Then, you wake up and you've gone viral overnight on social media or are suddenly being scouted for your soccer skills. Or "I can get through this. I can get through this." Which might spur you to feel you can cope with whatever comes your way.

Some people love these. They make boards and hang them on their walls: "Home is where the heart is," "I choose happiness," "I let go of all that no longer serves me," or "I deserve love." They feel like they're manifesting the things that they want in life, to be the person they dream of becoming. It feels satisfying, hopeful.

For others, these phrases seem too aspirational. Not realistic.

Some of my patients have told me that affirmations make them feel lousy. Like the goal isn't possible. To them, the phrase feels like they're lying to themselves. Over and over. Which, let's be honest, can make things worse. Self-gaslighting?

The point is to create a new pathway. For folks who've gone through trauma, one of the hardest things can be to dream that tomorrow would be different. That our mind could follow fresh paths.

> Iffirmations plant seeds of possibility.

And that's the amazing thing about the brain. Because of *neuroplasticity*, it's capable of forging new pathways. But think about it like a jungle. Your neural network is tangled and thick. Every time you think a thought or remember a memory, you travel down the neural pathway enforcing that connection. To shift anything, you hack at the weeds until there's a new way to travel. Your brain likes easy and familiar processes. It will preferentially choose the same path, even if it's not one you enjoy.

So, if your typical thinking process is "I am the worst. Nothing goes right for me. I don't deserve all the things," then that's the path that your brain chooses.

The goal of affirmations, or iffirmations, is to make new pathways. Ones that are optimistic, full of positive potential futures.

How can we take an affirmation and turn it into an iffirmation?

LET'S PRACTICE—IFFIRMATIONS

	AFFIRMATION	IFFIRMATION
Healing	I am healed.	What if I could heal?
Dreaming	Tomorrow will be better.	What if tomorrow will be better?
Wishing	I am enough.	What if I could consider I'm enough?

Check in with your body. How did each of these phrases make you feel? This is key.

Learn to notice what feels good for you. This can also change day to day, even hour to hour. Our brain is not static.

If the affirmation makes you feel hopeful—warm, tingling, dreamy, hugged—then you've got your answer. If it makes you feel uncertain, angry, agitated, or tense—then maybe it's not the right tool for you today.

What about the iffirmation? How did that feel?

If it still seems hard to believe, try "What if I could consider the possibility..." or "What if I can imagine a future when..."

Origin Story

Iffirmations aren't widely known. I first heard about them when I studied Havening. Some teachers used iffirmations while they practiced.

The coaches (Tony Burgess and Julie French) who developed these noted that lots of clients ask "what if"—to worry about the worst-case scenario. How often have each of us become anxious about the future, asking, "What if my flight is delayed?" "What if I can't pay my rent this month?" "What if this stomach problem is something really serious?" This pattern can keep our mind stuck in anxiety.

When you think about it, there's a protection mechanism involved. When the brain is trying to keep you safe from threats, when it considers the absolute worst possibilities, then it means you're more prepared for it should something happen. At least you've thought about it and won't be surprised.

This is what we call (in CBT) *catastrophizing*—thinking of the worst outcome.

The secret to iffirmations is using this natural process that our brain already does, but to turn it around. (A little opposite action, from DBT?) To ask *positive* "what if" questions.

Questions they suggest include:

- What if I can forgive myself and others?
- What if the universe is on my side?
- What if I am surrounded by opportunities and I just need to start noticing them?
- What if I can start to notice more of the great things in life?

You may notice that some questions on this list would take a gigantic leap of faith for the brain that's experienced trauma. It's a stretch to have a brain that's on the alert for danger to suddenly assume that "the universe is on my side." Especially when your lived experience hasn't made this seem true.

With a brain that's experienced trauma, you might start with "What if I could consider that the universe is on my side?" or "What if I could imagine myself believing in a time that this will be okay?" The extra distance into the future this creates might be more comfortable.

Daily Practice

An effective way to approach iffirmations is to build them into one's daily routine. Lots of people do this with affirmations. I think it can be equally powerful with the more tentative questions rather than the positive statements.

Here are a few that I've recommended for patients:

While you practice them, notice how your body feels. What nervous system state do they stir up? We want to create more time of the day when you're feeling calm and confident, so stick to the ones that help build these feelings.

- What if I was as kind to myself as I am to others?
- What if I told myself a different story about who I am?
- What if I deserve good things?
- What if I am enough?
- What if I can get through this?

Mental Flexibility

We search for more enjoyable pathways for your brain, which is different for every person.

As a physician therapist, I try to help a patient achieve mental flexibility. Think about that brain jungle full of tangled neural trees—hacking alternative paths means you can explore new, safer territory. You don't continue to go down the path toward negative, self-harming thoughts and behaviors every time. You don't have to tread the path toward a stress response—either the high-tone activated one or the low-tone disconnect.

It leaves these as two feasible options, out of many others. We all need to run away or fight off genuine threats. But the problem is that, especially after trauma, our brain locks into the path of alarm. So that, while the danger is only one of many possibilities, the brain reacts as if the threat is certain.

Iffirmations help create the flexibility in this response.

It takes practice. These pathways toward stress become like a reflex. You're in a situation in the present time—let's imagine the sound of a speeding car, as an example. If you've been in a car accident in the past, this sound might be triggering. So, the pathway tells your brain it's unsafe, and your body wants to run away.

This reaction shows up in your body as tense muscles, heart pounding—all the physical sensations that mean you're on high alert. You may get restless legs and move away from the sound.

Now, imagine that you hear the car but with more mental flexibility. Cue iffirmations:

- What if the car is far away?
- What if the car is on the other side of the road?
- What if the car just sounds loud because it's missing a muffler?

You get the point.

Of course, many talk therapy techniques create mental flexibility. Those you can remember, don't self-gaslight, and don't add to the burden of shame are the ones I find the most useful.

When you read through this chapter, which ideas did you notice helped your nervous system get more calm? Which were activating? Which made you bored, where you didn't have any interest?

Remember, the first step is noticing. The next step is shifting. You're getting more and more ideas on how to shift.

This is how you build your toolkit.

CHAPTER 25

Community

Trauma doesn't happen in a vacuum; it happens in relation with other people. Healing happens the same way.

One of the biggest misconceptions about trauma is that it's like a giant wound you need to clean up yourself. First, it's not a wound. You're not broken. Your body is doing exactly what it is designed to do. It thinks it's protecting you from suffering. So, trauma is more like thick armor. But it slows you down from doing the things you truly want in life. When you find other ways of protecting yourself, you don't need it to be so heavy. Second, it's not something easily carried or resolved alone.

Trauma happens in a context: a time, a place, and a society. Sometimes horrible actions are tolerated when people have power or privilege; society protects abusers more than the people they hurt. Think of the history of Salem, when townsfolk accused women they didn't like of being witches. Or look at modern-day Hollywood. Communities protect harmful teachers, coaches, or religious leaders. Racist practices are encoded in laws and policies.

Related to ancestral traumas that haven't healed, we end up with cultures that express trauma through cycles of violence and collective dissociation. We see this shutting-down effect in policy-makers hoping that the climate emergency will go away, despite the evidence that it won't unless we make massive changes. We use entertainment (sports, music) to bond with each other, but getting too wrapped up in it can be dissociative. Many people use drugs or gaming to switch off their overthinking brain.

A concept that might be unfamiliar is *decolonizing*. The best primers on this include the stunning *Braiding Sweetgrass* by Robin Wall Kimmerer or the books I mentioned in Chapter 6, *Decolonizing Trauma Work* by Renee Linklater and *Decolonizing Methodologies* (with a research focus) by Linda Tuhiwai Smith.

A lot of the traumas that we face in modern times have to do with structures that are counter to our Indigenous ways of knowing and being. I say "our" because it's not only First Nations people of the Americas (and globally) who have land-based and collectivist traditions. My Ukrainian ancestors had them. My Scottish ancestors also had them. Up to two hundred years ago, people lived in close-knit villages and looked after one another. This isn't something we innately know how to do anymore.

In all contexts, Indigenous people were harmed by European invaders willing to murder for land and resources. Such colonized actions continue today, including in the harm caused by health care (forced sterilizations, apprehending children, making false assumptions). Decolonization means that we actively consider the harms to the original people who were first on these lands and consider how they might co-create a return to more natural and connected ways.

Individual ways of innovating are insufficient to meet the challenges of modern times. This is because issues are complex, and they need contributions from different perspectives to solve these problems. These larger-scale traumas, like inequity and environmental issues, need a hive mind. I say "hive" deliberately, because we have the capacity to function like a group of bees that are cross-pollinating and working together for the greater good.

In *The Extended Mind*, Annie Murphy Paul describes how to create a group mind through:

- Synchrony—when we move together in unison, or create things that are the same, it makes us feel cohesive. We become better collaborators and co-conspirators. *I love learning new crafts in a group, from Ukrainian egg painting to "paint nights" with the same canvas model.*
- Shared physiology—when we enter a high activation state together, through either physical movement or emotion, it makes us feel we're working together. *A few of my friends do triathlon competitions together.*

- Shared attention—this can be as simple as looking in the same direction, but when we attune to the same thing, we get a sense of similar experience. This can include learning something together or having an emotional experience together. *Imagine people all watching a rocket fly into space or viewing a football game.*
- Rituals—from eating lunch in the cafeteria to having a ceremony to celebrate an occasion. An expectation of a group activity creates anticipation and cohesion. *Think of a sales group that goes out for dinner to celebrate a deal or college friends who go to a club to dance.*

How can we create a group scenario that is trauma-informed and follows these practices so the group feels bonded? In Radha Agrawal's book *Belong*, where she writes about creating community and one thing she did herself was start morning dance parties she calls Daybreakers. I wish there were Daybreakers in my city!

LET'S PRACTICE—SYNC

First, you want to create a common purpose. What is something that a hypothetical group wants to do?

Let's imagine that the group wants to invite members to explore different healing activities.

They might try a yoga class or have a spoken-word night. There might be an ecstatic dance party. Any practices that could be performed together.

So, tonight, this group will explore mindful eating.

Their joint activity is something simple, like food prep. Chopping vegetables, making juice, baking cookies. To really cement the feeling of cohesion, they would do something else in synchrony.

What about singing something as they prepare?

This works better if the song brings out an emotional response, then you get the "physiological synchrony" as well. If not, being busy in the kitchen is probably enough to get the heart rate up enough to rouse the body.

Learning something together is part of the work of the team. Let's say each community member researches a topic and they share with the group what they studied. For this evening session, they'd learn how to smell every morsel and examine the texture—blindfolding may add fun.

Assuming everybody eats the meal together, chewing slowly, savoring each bite, this would provide the shared attention. If they're sharing a lesson and their food, it's a collective experience on many levels.

Circles

I've already mentioned a practice through an Indigenous healing workshop at the University of British Columbia that was meaningful and fun—circle dancing. It got me thinking about how many communal activities we have lost (or forcefully buried) in modern times that could heal us from traumatic experiences.

During the workshop, the instructor led us through six different dances, originating from different countries across the world. We stood in a circle and moved in unison. Some dances were very complex, requiring that we hold hands or weave around like a giant snake. There was a ton of laughter—it felt joyful and freeing. You could sense the way that the group felt about each other changed after we danced together. In modern times, DJs create communal rhythmic experiences, using beat drops or working to hype up the crowd.

Assets

The Tamarack Institute in Canada speaks about strength-based community work and collective impact. In one of their toolkits, they describe how "the community narrative is the story that citizens tell each other about living and working [together]." Part of the story is statistics, like the ages and other demographics of the people who are in the community. Other pieces to the story include shared history and the meaning that persists in the present. Resources and skills within the collective are another piece of that story.

The Tamarack Institute developed an *asset inventory tool* so that a community can discover more information about which resources exist to be shared and those that need to be developed. Assets can include natural ones (without having a sense of ownership but more to be in relationship with the natural environment), physical structures (like buildings or parks), jobs or businesses, or services. Also, social assets like traditions and beliefs, as well as whether people will work together toward common goals. The word "asset" sounds like it's commodifying the items so there needs to be conscious attention to prevent this—we are so conditioned in Western culture around capitalism.

When I think about both the circle dances and the strengths within communities, I think of some of my refugee patients. When trauma is stuck in their body, there may have been a traditional ceremony in their country of origin that would have shifted their nervous system into a calm and connected state. Whether that was an aged-based ritual, thinking about how their community dances or sings together, or wearing traditional clothes that connected them to their ancestors. When I do guided imagery work with refugee patients, these concepts often create safe spaces and invoke memories of experiences separate from trauma.

Start Small

I often recommend a tool called "10 percent solutions." Instead of trying to accomplish a task or goal all at once, which can be overwhelming, try to get 10 percent of the way. Communities can do the same. Taking small steps to move in the direction that creates safer spaces and less opportunity for suffering isn't something that shifts overnight. We can transition slowly by moving 10 percent at a time. This will seem more manageable and then the group won't get stuck in an overwhelmed state.

Groups can also freeze and flood.

In real life, this would look like a neighborhood wanting to make the street safer for kids to play. It can feel daunting to think of everything that needs done. So, a "10 percent solution" might be to put up a sign that says to slow down. Or to call the city to make sure all the streetlamps work. Or start with a single event like a giant game (my neighbors do egg hunts at Easter and have a street-wide garage sale).

One thing that has been a challenge in group work is having polarized beliefs about an issue. Whether it's how to manage public health during a pandemic, or defining priorities with a limited budget, certain voices become dominant, and this can lead to frustration. Racism and sexism often play a role. One of the key strategies that I've learned in creating safer dialogue is to focus on shared values, even if they're not in the same order of priority. By acknowledging and agreeing on these values, conversation is possible on any issue, no matter how controversial or divided.

Here's an Example

One of the greatest jobs I've had in my career so far has been working with community members in groups that we called the "Solutions Studio." I had been studying *social innovation labs,* where people joined to solve complex challenges in small groups. This felt like a fantastic idea for a health clinic, since problems don't seem so massive if we tackle them together. And the patients are the experts on their own problems and dream up solutions out of necessity.

The first step was deciding on a shared priority. I deliberately invited groups of people who had a common lived experience. The first group had mobility challenges. The next group was dealing with chronic pain. A third group had experienced trauma and wanted to create a safer experience when accessing their health care.

Each group started by designing an *empathy map,* by considering a generic story of a person who might deal with a similar challenge (this way, no one had to share their personal experience if they didn't feel comfortable). On the empathy map, they debated the feelings a person might have in the context of the challenge—what barriers they might face and what resources they might have. We talked about "pain points" in the system and tasks they had to accomplish to reach their goals. After this exercise, the group generally felt they had a shared understanding of the problem.

DESIGN THINKING

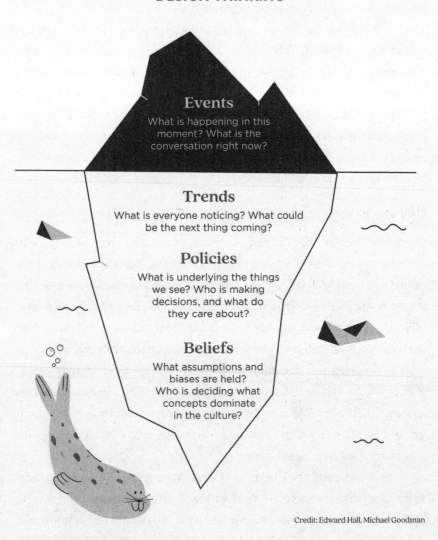

Events
What is happening in this
moment? What is the
conversation right now?

Trends
What is everyone noticing? What could
be the next thing coming?

Policies
What is underlying the things
we see? Who is making
decisions, and what do
they care about?

Beliefs
What assumptions and
biases are held?
Who is deciding what
concepts dominate
in the culture?

Credit: Edward Hall, Michael Goodman

Our next step was to look at the *iceberg model of systems-change*. The tip of the iceberg is what you see in public discussions, social media, stories in the news, and "word on the street" (this can include trending topics, current events, or memes).

The layer under this, what you can't always see, is the policies and infrastructure that create the challenge. For the group dealing with mobility issues, "pain points" included transportation and the building code not ensuring accessible entrances. For the group that was experiencing chronic pain, it was a sense of being dismissed. For the folks experiencing trauma, they wanted transparent expectations for patients coming to the clinic (from the staff).

Underneath, at the bottom of the iceberg model, are the assumptions that people make. Society has biases about pain, or people with disability, or those who've been through trauma (or someone facing all three issues).

The last step was for the group to generate solutions. It was incredible to witness and participate in this part of the session. Creative ideas were flying, enthusiasm was shared, and there was a spirited belief that change was possible. The mobility group secured a grant to create a promotional video demonstrating the challenges of getting around the city, which was an interesting and practical activity to share. They learned new skills and had a concrete tool to do their own advocacy. The chronic pain group created a support meeting for men that connected every week, led by a social worker who understood their challenges. They also asked for a space to make lots of noise to distract themselves from pain, so they were offered times to use the health center's music room. The group who had been through trauma presented their charter of rights to the leadership team at the health center to see if their lived experience could influence the treatment of patients. This is something people facing homelessness had constructed, so we built on a solution already created in a different, but related, community.

This experience taught me something that I suspected: if you create an opportunity for groups to thrive, they can often solve their own complex challenges. It can be very empowering for people who are entering a system designed with their vulnerabilities in mind instead of their strengths to flip the hierarchy. To show that they have power to make change, and that their vulnerabilities give them the knowledge, experience, and sometimes tools to make that happen.

Stories

We mentioned the community story. Many groups who deal with people who've been through traumatic experiences focus on *storytelling*. This is another practice that humans have been using since ancient times. We pass traditional wisdom through story and metaphor.

There's a free online course on narrative practice offered by an Aboriginal group in Australia at the Dulwich Centre. In the book *Aboriginal Narrative Practice*, they outlined some tools that they described online. One of them is to create a tree of life focusing on:

- the roots, which include ancestors and traditions
- the ground of everyday life
- the trunk of values and qualities
- the branches of hopes and dreams
- the leaves of special connections
- the fruits of the gifts that have been given

Of the many narrative practices that they describe, another is the *listening team*. People gather and decide on a theme to discuss, and a listening team sits behind the group, keeping notes and paying attention. At a break in the conversation, the listening team enters the middle of the circle and reflects on what they had heard. This practice often brings a sense of validation and pride, especially if the group had survived tremendous challenges.

Indigenous groups throughout the world have been creating local approaches to collective trauma. Because so many of them faced genocide by settler colonialism, there is a great deal of generational trauma to work through. They still hold a lot of this trauma in the body, which can show up as fight-or-flight or freeze energy states of individuals and of groups. It's one reason there's a history of substance use and addiction in some modern communities—to numb the pain of the past and the ongoing problems colonialism still creates in their families.

I've learned of theater programs in the New Zealand Māori, a resurgence of traditional dance among Hawaiians, and Indigenous healing practices in Canada (like the sweat lodge and the Sundance). The herbal medicines related to mental health are only a small fraction of what they know throughout the world. Many Indigenous peoples have a long relationship with plants, as well as rituals that lead to transformational, trancelike states. In modern times, we are only starting to understand how deeply healing these practices are. Mourn what has been lost while celebrating what is saved.

Here's an Example

As somebody who fought cancer at a young age, Lara was eager to join a *digital storytelling* project. She wanted to describe everything she'd been through—not to sugarcoat her experiences, but to let people know that it's possible to get through them.

It was hard sifting through old photographs of when she had lost her hair, how skinny she was, and seeing her parents by her bedside. Now that her dad was gone, photos of him always make her cry. She'll always wonder if it was the stress of her illness that was too much for him. As immigrants, they had their hopes pinned on her future. When it seemed like she might not have one, her whole family seemed to be ill. This was the story she wanted to tell. Even though Lara had survived cancer, her family had changed forever.

The person running the project showed participants how to tell a story in three minutes. Lara practiced so that she could say it without getting too emotional. After the recording, she shocked herself at how professional it sounded. They chose photographs or artwork to match each of the aspects of her story that she told. She bonded with the other participants, since everyone shared such profound stories, and they often went out for a coffee when they finished in the studio.

The team screened their stories on the campus of the medical school. All the storytellers were treated like royalty. Lara's video was met with thunderous applause. She felt awkward and proud, feeling the audience had truly seen her.

There is a fascinating practice called *constellations work*—both family constellations and systems constellations. Organizers represent family members or pieces of the system with either humans to "act" (pose) or with objects (like Lego pieces). The people involved then use their intuition to determine how each of these pieces move.

This kind of work helps us discover more about our future. Learning about the dynamics of each participant in the story helps us see "the bigger picture." When we consider the whole system, when we lean into our intuition, when we consider our collective future—this heals communities.

Our work together is to create a world where all systems: individual bodies, families, communities, and the ecosystem experience less trauma. And heal together. This is how we nurture our path to post-traumatic growth.

EXTRAS

CHAPTER 26

Policies

We could prevent trauma from a systemic level by supporting policies that reduce the conditions that contribute to it. If you're in a position of leadership, of influencing decisions, or even if you have the power to vote—you can catalyze change.

Income

A universal basic income (a.k.a. UBI: financial support, with no requirements or conditions, given to every citizen by their government) or guaranteed income (provided to those living in poverty) would give people a reliable foundation when they have no ability to work because of ill health or social circumstances. This income would need to be above the poverty line and allow for emergency contingencies because there are too many "working poor" and people living precariously. We saw firsthand during the COVID-19 pandemic just how fragile income can be, and many countries, like Canada, provided monthly financial aid to their citizens in need. We cannot let the obscenely wealthy escape taxation, which would easily cover such costs. There's a more recent turning toward guaranteed income that acknowledges inequity. People with mental or physical health conditions face this reality every day.

> Have there been any research trials in your country
> around a guaranteed minimum income?
> How might we advocate for more pilot studies
> and a long-term feasibility plan?

Universal Care

Besides income assurance, we need to support policies and practices that provide basic health care for all. It's ludicrous when only the rich can afford health care. Governments should provide for physical health services—but also mental health, vision care, dental care, pharmaceuticals and vitamins, rehab after surgery or stroke, palliative care at the end of life, and more. Western medicine is not the only worthy paradigm—we know the benefits from nutrition and lifestyle medicine, cultural medical practices (Ayurveda, Traditional Chinese Medicine), and plant medicines—and we should allow people to choose their healing path.

> How might we advocate for the broadest coverage of
> health care where you live?
> How might we help people understand that we aren't
> healthy as a community until all of us are healthy?

Parenting

We should have accessible, culturally appropriate parenting classes representing different stages of life. Additional options should be available for people on both sides of adoption, since there are special considerations in this scenario. Likewise, parenting support groups should exist, and with diverse facilitators and experts. We can create ways for parents to share information and childcare among themselves—spending time together and parenting alongside one another.

> How might we provide parents with the best
> support for success in giving their kids a (physically,
> emotionally, and socially) safe environment?
> What else could be done to prevent adverse
> childhood experiences?

Anti-oppression

All organizations and professionals should have policies in place to prevent structural discrimination. We all have biases in our subconscious mind, so the more support that is written out in policy form, the better chance we have to overcome these. Rania El Mugammar outlines how to facilitate *anti-oppression work*—she calls it "designing for liberation." In her perspective, *equality* means giving everyone the same thing, *equity* means giving everyone what they need, and anti-oppression work entails taking down the barriers that lead to the inequity. Rania clarifies that those with the most privilege have more responsibility to take the biggest risks in advocating for all others. Lawyer Valarie Kaur advocates a Love Revolution—her book *See No Stranger* and her TED Talk speak to reclamation of love as a public ethic.

> Beyond having committees around diversity and inclusion,
> what other concrete actions could your organizations and
> community do to shift the power balance?
> How can group processes lay a path to shift attitudes,
> increase knowledge, and build skills in
> education and evaluation?

Crisis Plan

We need new emergency services where we dispatch mental health support for social crises to prevent accidents, deaths, and arrests. At baseline, we need all first responders to be trauma-informed, because many of the situations they're attending will require care based on equity and safety. We've seen problems, even violence, in having police officers attend all distress calls—it's unfair to communities and to police. Cheri Maples, a police officer and meditation teacher, co-founded the Center for Mindfulness and Justice, helping others identify their unconscious biases. Resmaa Menakem's book *My Grandmother's Hands* focuses on three separate streams of practice: for Black bodies, for white bodies, and for police.

> How could the first responders in your neighborhood
> be prepared to attend to psychological distress?
> How might we uncover novel ways of attending a crisis,
> based on justice and accountability?

Collaboration

Whenever we change policies or laws, there needs to be meaningful consultation and input from the communities who will be affected. We should provide information they require in an understandable format and in their languages. There should be ways for everybody to express their perspective, not just leaders who typically voice the opinion of the dominant viewpoint. Cultural brokers, chosen by the community, could be a representative voice—as they could gather the consensus and alternative ideas in confidence and collaboration.

> How might we advocate for implementing an advisory
> council (a consultation of clients or citizens) in
> public and private organizations?
> How might we ensure representation of the
> quieter voices of our community in decisions?

Metrics

We can't change what we don't see. Measuring the impact of race or gender on health will show where discrimination still exists. Likewise, before they conducted studies on adverse childhood experiences, we didn't know how they impact people in later life. More research like this needs to take place—to measure and acknowledge problems so that we can actively change them. To avoid retraumatizing people with the information, we would implement ethical and anti-oppressive data collection.

> What kind of information might help drive
> change where you live?
> How could those with resources collect information
> and co-create research strategy with mutual benefit?

CHAPTER 27

Psych First Aid

Most of us have heard of physical first aid—you check if someone is breathing and if they have a pulse. But what about psychological first aid? Can someone who's not a therapist intervene and help? Could you prevent PTSD by offering appropriate support during a crisis?

Absolutely—you can.

In the event of a major emergency, it's likely that public services including ambulances and firetrucks will be on scene shortly. Most people pay attention to physical injuries and forget psychological trauma. I took an online course in psychological first aid from Johns Hopkins; some of the following ideas come from those teachings. Others came from World Health Organization documents and other disaster management guidelines.

The effects of dangerous situations are influenced by the nature and severity of the event, its meaning, prior (including childhood) trauma, age at occurrence, cultural factors, available supports, and baseline health status.

STEP ONE: SCREEN

Physical Check

- ❐ Look for immediate ongoing danger risks and clear the area.
- ❐ Consider phoning an ambulance right away if injury is obvious.
- ❐ If they're speaking, this means that airway and pulse are present.
- ❐ If they're unconscious, establish heart and breathing rate (if you know how).

☐ If there's no pulse, establish compression-only CPR (take a class if you haven't learned yet).

☐ Look for major injuries or bleeding, try to splint (hold in place, apply pressure to wound).

☐ See if there are any signs of stroke, heart attack, breaks, or internal bleeding.

☐ Stay out of the way of first responders or rescue crews.

☐ Watch out for unaccompanied children or people with disabilities who need quick intervention.

Psychological Check

☐ Trauma can happen to both brain and body after a natural disaster or similarly dangerous violent event.

☐ If it looks like somebody needs assistance, always check in with your own nervous system—are you able to help them stay calm? Even if your own body is in fight, flight, or freeze—you might still be in the Window of Tolerance where you can help.

☐ Is anybody in immediate psychological danger? Who could you contact? Consider family members, care team, mental health outreach, trusted community leaders, or police. Get consent first, if possible.

☐ If someone is in immediate danger to themselves or others, this is a psychiatric emergency and they need urgent medical attention.

☐ Look for people who seem confused and disoriented. Helping to ground them in safety can shift their nervous system. If they remain in shock, they need medical attention.

☐ Ask for consent from the person at risk before any intervention. Don't assume the best way to keep them safe. This is especially true of any physical touch and sometimes even eye contact.

☐ Remember, police and authority figures are not always trusted and appropriate for everyone (especially for Black and Indigenous people, members of the LGBTQIA2S+ community, and those from places who experienced past disasters but felt abandoned).

STEP TWO: LISTEN

☐ Let them know you're willing to listen if they want to talk, or just be with them if they're feeling nervous or anxious. A calm presence can make an enormous difference in these moments, since isolation is one aspect of an event that creates the trauma response.

☐ Offer companionship but as an invitation, not an expectation. "I'm happy to sit here with you, if that's something you'd like, but also able to give you space if you prefer that."

☐ You might need a translator, interpreter, or cultural support person to help. Follow principles of respect, dignity, and confidentiality at all times.

☐ Ground them in the moment, something like "You're not alone, and I'm here with you right here, right now," in a soft, slow tone of voice.

☐ You don't necessarily want to encourage them to talk about the details of the event. As you now know, every time you tell the story, the pathway toward the memory and those details gets stronger. Debriefing after an experience does not help prevent PTSD.

☐ Instead, find something out about who they are and what resources they might have available (safe places or people) or what might be missing (objects or loved ones) where you could help with a search. Ensure they have essential medical devices (hearing aids, glasses, mobility aids, medications, service animals) and prescription medicines.

☐ Offer compassionate, nonjudgmental words in response to anything they say that sounds stressful. Phrases like "That sounds really hard, thank you for sharing," or "I'm so sorry this happened to you, and I'm glad that you are safe now" can keep them in the present moment while showing that you're actively listening.

☐ Avoid any assumptions if you feel compelled to reassure them: they may *not* be glad to have survived if they have lost family members, they may *not* feel strong enough to get through it, they may *not* believe it happened for a reason.

❏ Some people prefer validation from sharing their story. It's sometimes helpful to be heard and to know that your suffering mattered and that others care. If a survivor insists on telling those details, decide about whether there's a risk of your own *vicarious trauma* (psychological distress from hearing a story secondhand) or if you can safely provide support.

❏ If it's not something you're comfortable hearing, set the boundary with compassion. Something like "I wish I was an expert in mental health, and I could help better with your distress. I'm able to sit here with you until we can try to connect you with an expert who'll be able to do that."

❏ Remind them to consider staying away from news and social media—they may be inclined to absorb all the details to get questions answered, but this might be harmful in the long run.

❏ Be clear about what you are able to do; avoid relaying any information that's still uncertain (causing false hope or unnecessary anguish) and don't provide any reassurance or promises that might not be possible.

❏ If they prefer not to speak at all, offering a simple video game on your phone or something monotonous to do with their hands (fidget toys) could be helpful.

STEP THREE: CONNECT

❏ You can counteract the trauma response by repeating their words back to them in a gentle voice. It lets them know their words matter and are understood, and your calm voice helps their nervous system mirror yours.

❏ Don't try to solve all of their immediate problems, but ask if there is something they'd like you to help with.

❐ If they are open to it, offer a point of contact—a hand on their shoulder, knee, or holding theirs might be reassuring.

❐ All emotions are welcome. Grief, anger, frustration, sadness. If you feel you can manage what's coming up, you might allow them to express whatever they feel without trying to rush them through their emotions.

❐ You might let them know that they might have difficulties with sleep, appetite, and being around other people in the short term—these are normal responses to danger, based on our threatened signals in the brain.

    ○ "Your body has been working really hard to protect you, so you might struggle with sleeping."

    ○ "You have been in survival mode, so all these reactions are very normal."

    ○ "It takes time for your body, mind, and spirit to accept that you've survived this threat."

❐ Don't make these reactions seem like they're wrong or strange (avoid words like *symptoms* or *disorder*).

❐ Focus on how they are strong and survived rather than any perceived weakness or disability (if they have one, they're still competent at many things).

STEP FOUR: RESOURCE

❐ Be on the lookout for mental health symptoms like total hopelessness, delusions or hallucinations, or significant disorientation. Any of these situations might need professional help.

❐ Let them know that surviving significant events doesn't always lead to PTSD. The key is knowing they aren't alone and there's no ongoing threat (if that is true).

❐ If you know somatic tools that you'd feel comfortable sharing, any of Havening, TRE, or EFT could be helpful in preventing the wiring of the brain toward trauma pathways (this is not evidence-based, but unlikely to be harmful). The Trauma Tapping Technique was developed to help in disaster situations and is easy to learn online or through *Trauma Tapping Technique* by Gunilla Hamne and Ulf Sandström.

❏ Preliminary research shows that suggesting they share their emotions using "what's one word you want to say or whisper" could be a helpful intervention.

❏ Writing might also be helpful—structured narratives that might invoke meaning, provide context, and question faulty assumptions that might be forming.

❏ Remind people they have a choice to leave a setting that could continue to cause harm, while keeping in mind cultural (honorbound) or social (financial resources or ties of children) reasons they may not want to leave. Let them know you'll support them in any instance.

❏ If children are at risk, this requires a call to Child Protective Services. Leave this to the experts but let them know what you've witnessed or heard. This involvement is not always straightforward, as historical harms have happened from their presence (forced apprehension of Black, Latino, and Indigenous children or from people who use drugs) and there may be valid mistrust.

❏ Offer, to the best of your ability, to help them find resources they might need.
  - "Should I look for water? Or clean clothing?"
  - "Is there anyone we could call to help?"

❏ There might be services that can take over assistance, but community support is just as valid. Do they have friends and neighbors? What's your own comfort zone around what you can do?

❏ Social services, distress lines, activist or advocacy groups, nonprofits, employee benefit plans, social workers, religious affiliates, counselors, therapists, psychologists, survivor support services, emergency shelters, general physicians, grief groups, and psychiatrists can all be helpful for a variety of needs.

❐ Help them make a list of their preferred support system. A Wellness Recovery Action Plan (WRAP) is something that can be done without professional guidance—the WRAP for trauma is a reasonably priced tool.

LET'S PRACTICE—WRITE A WRAP PLAN

---

1. List wellness tools

Common wellness tools include talking to someone who validates you, stress reduction exercises, guided imagery, extra rest, listing options, appreciating something, listening to music.

Less common wellness tools include sucking your thumb, getting in the shower with all your clothes still on, hitting pillows, writing what bothers you and tearing it up, coloring.

2. Write out your daily maintenance plan

Food and drink intake, who and what to avoid, activities, prevention plans

3. List triggers

Different for everyone and for every situation. Common ones include dates, places, sensory experiences, communication styles, intimacy, noises, visuals.

4. Early warning signs

These are different for everyone, but it's best to try to notice when heavy emotions are sneaking up. Some ideas: nightmares, worrying, hopelessness, apathy, cravings, avoiding the phone, change in eating patterns, feeling rejected, nothing to look forward to, spending time with the wrong people

5. Activities for triggers and early signs

These are ideas for what might prevent you from going from "triggered" to "traumatized." Some suggestions: get outside, wear cheerful clothes, meet friends, play music, ask for help, nap, watch movies.

6. Time to take action

What are the indicators that things are not going well? It could be flashbacks, thoughts of self-harm, being oversensitive, substance use, dissociation, anger, lack of self-care, avoiding everyone, self-loathing, being afraid of everything, feeling undeserving or guilty.

7. Emergency planning

Create a personal list for psychological emergency plans. Consider: have someone come stay with you, methods to prevent self-harm (safely store medications or weapons), take time off work, try breath work or meditation, get a massage, visit your therapist, use calming self-talk, exercise, seek validation, distract through entertainment or sports, develop new routines, or engage in slow body-based relaxation practices.

8. Signs others need to take over

How do you know when you're being yourself or not—naming characteristics that are not typical for you (mood swings, self-destructive choices, agitated pacing, violence, not getting out of bed are some examples)—then naming five people (which can be caregivers) to support. Also name people you don't want involved, medications that do or don't work for you, things you want your supporters to try, places you might go for respite (hospitals do not always work for people), and the signs that you're back to your usual self so that your supporters can gently back away.

9. Postcrisis planning

Includes: comfortable place to recover, things you might need help with when reintegrating, what to avoid, any results (financial, legal, social, employment) that you must deal with, and resting

STEP FIVE: REFLECT

- ❏ Be clear about your own availability for follow-up.
- ❏ Take some time to process your own feelings about it all.
- ❏ Think about it from first-, second- (survivor), and third-person perspectives.

❏ Consider writing some notes for yourself about your thoughts, your emotions, and your reactions. Sometimes the crisis is hard to remember, as our cognitive brain goes offline. Journaling could help in testimony, in filling in gaps for the survivor, or in your own analysis. I like to write poetry in these kinds of situations.

❏ Do you have any survivor guilt? Any shame in your responses? How can you work through that?

❏ Could it help to mark the anniversary of the event with a ritual? There might be an ongoing connection between survivors and responders.

❏ Be vigilant for the signs of vicarious (secondary) trauma, compassion fatigue, or burnout. Feeling cynical or hopeless, exhausted or dissociated, or needing to step away are signs you need some time to recover your own resilience.

❏ *Vicarious resilience* is possible. Witnessing the recovery, the strength, and the post-traumatic growth of others can improve our own mental health.

CHAPTER 28

Finding a Therapist

It's sometimes challenging to find a therapist. Even if you have the resources, whether paying for it yourself or through a work assistance plan, or if there are free public services, you have to ensure it's a good fit. A therapist that doesn't have the same values or outlook can do harm, causing *medical trauma*.

You might find a therapist through word of mouth, like asking on social media (people may prefer to text or private-message with personal information). Ask friends for references, while noting that reviews online are dominated by the most unsatisfied clients, so they're often biased.

Some of the large psychological businesses—I won't name the ones that are culprits right now, since it's likely to change—don't pay their therapists well. It might mean they're reasonably priced—but the therapists may not have good qualifications, or they might be overworked and burned out. The enterprise might have unsafe professional practices, and the company could use your information in ways you might not consider. Many newer apps and sites ask for monthly subscription fees. Check reviews and testimonials to ensure you'll get what you're paying for (emergency visits, weekly sessions, reaching someone—not an AI bot—by text, or virtual resources).

Some programs have charitable paths to find a therapist for little or no cost. Many therapists will take a sliding scale—adjusting their fee to your income and capacity.

The first session is a chance to learn and decide if each wants to continue the therapeutic relationship. So, you're interviewing them just as much as they're interviewing you. It used to be the case that this session was free, but that's happening less often. If you don't have coverage, advocate for an exception or ask if there's a flexible payment scheme.

Here are some questions to consider. Bring a pen and notebook or write these (with the answers) on a phone or tablet.

If it's accessible (not everyone notices instinct signals if their body has learned to ignore them), a "gut instinct" about somebody can be the best way to decide.

Questions to consider might include:

- Their background, philosophy about trauma, and qualifications (are they a clinical social worker, psychologist, medical doctor or osteopath, nurse practitioner, or coach?)
- They may be comfortable sharing their religious background, if they have children, or their political affiliation, if this matters a lot to you.
- The type of therapies they practice (even if you don't know the ones they mention, you can ask for more details or look them up once you're home to see if it's something that interests you)
- If they have a specialty (for example, some therapists enjoy working with certain communities or have extra training with an issue such as addiction, eating, grief, or trauma)
- Their experience of working with the issues you're wanting to discuss
- Their experience of working with any communities that you identify with, whether that's race- or culture-based, sexuality or gender, neurodiversity, or anything else
- How long it will take you to get an appointment and how often you'd expect to be seen? (It might be weekly to start, then move to every two or four weeks when things are more stable.)
- Can they do virtual care, and can you make online bookings or cancellations?
- How does payment work, do they have a sliding scale, and can they direct-bill an employer program or insurance?
- What does the space look and feel like (some rooms have pillows, weighted blankets, choice of scents or lighting)?

- The length of a typical session
- What happens if you miss a session?
- What happens if they miss a session (for example, if they charge you for a missed time, would they do the same in return with a free session if they cancel)?
- Who has access to their records and their diagnosis, including your personal details?
- How do they decide when you no longer need therapy? (You don't want to be paying someone for life.)

After the initial meeting, you might have an idea if it's a good match. The purpose is to find a caring, compassionate supporter to help you navigate healing.

Do they seem to respect your ideas? Do they listen? Do they explain what they're thinking? Are they good communicators? Does it seem like they care? Do you have a sense they might help?

When someone has experienced trauma, trust can take time to establish. If you don't feel ready to trust them with your big emotions or private stories, that is entirely up to you. We should all be willing to "move at the speed of trust."

It might be awkward to refuse a second appointment. Ways to end such a session could be a phrase like, "I appreciate your time. It was nice learning more about your practice, but I don't think it's a great fit for me. I'll perhaps send people your way that might be a better match." You can also be less committal: "Thanks for this. I'm still considering other options, so I'll be in touch."

Once you've begun therapy, there's a power dynamic in the relationship that could feel uncomfortable at first. When you have been through trauma, authority figures and professionals might not feel safe. Acknowledge this (to yourself, or potentially to them) and notice if this change is part of the therapy process. When you have had control taken from you, these relationships with an inherent power differential can be hard to establish.

Keep in mind that the "connected" nervous system may not be available to you when you first explore therapy. This means that your gut instinct may be "offline," and you might even gravitate to familiar patterns that might cause you further harm. Even though most therapists do their best to avoid it, we are not perfect—we can gaslight, we have racist and other biases, and we make mistakes. The therapy room might be the first environment where you can draw boundaries, where you can express your true feelings. Make sure this feels supported.

If you agree to a virtual session, make sure the connection complies with information privacy laws (secure, not recorded, password protected). Make sure that your setting feels safe and that you can establish privacy away from partners or children (headphones help, but they'll still hear your voice, so they aren't ideal and may prevent honest expression).

One of the most effective interventions that all therapists can do is "Feedback Informed Treatment," a term coined and researched by Scott D. Miller. This means the therapist asks what worked and didn't work during the session. If they're truly listening and shifting their style, you'll know they're paying attention and trying their best.

We are not the experts on your context and experience. You are.

CHAPTER 29

Safer Spaces

How might we create safer spaces outside the home? For people who've experienced trauma, no place is truly safe because your brain perceives danger. Likewise, we cannot scrub colonialism and ingrained prejudice from our mind. The idea of "safer" spaces is that we can try to create the conditions for safety, provide education about these natural responses to more and more people, and try to lower the risk of further harm for everyone.

> No one should face racism, discrimination, cruelty, and
> harassment anywhere.
> There should be dignity, mutual respect, accountability, empathy,
> and equity in all spaces.

There is pushback against trauma-informed training as protecting those who benefit from existing systems. Those with privilege might experience trauma with the loss of their authority, autonomy, entitlements, and social position. Part of being trauma-informed means examining these possibilities.

I don't intend for these suggestions to be prescriptive, as that can maintain the balance of power. Trauma is culturally, contextually, and politically informed. We subconsciously protect those with similar personal background and social position. I write this in the Global North, by and for those who benefit from historical and structural violence. My goal is to contribute to a more complex conversation about trauma that welcomes critique and paradox. I am complicit in many traumatic environments and claim no moral high ground. What I offer is curiosity and flexibility, along with a willingness to learn and grow.

When we have leisure time, we seek experiences with like-minded people. These can be hobbies, sports, and community groups. It might also be activist spaces—the narrower the focus, the more likely you are to feel kinship (think: Black trans women or Latinx vegans). These might be the safest places possible, especially something like an official "safe place" for queer folks. But they can also be a further source of vicarious (secondhand) pain— I've heard this story from people who attend 12-step programs that get triggered listening to difficult (and familiar) stories at meetings.

School, work, and leisure environments can be a source of trauma, from a lot of directions:

- Being stuck in a hierarchical (power at the top) structure that ignores or distorts your authentic voice
- Microaggressions about your ethnic background (like people wanting to touch your hair or telling you that your home-cooked food smells)
- Anxiety about performance that stirs up "not good enough" feelings
- Feeling helpless or hopeless
- Feeling abandoned or neglected, which might bring up childhood issues
- Bullying or cliques

In creating "Safer Spaces," acknowledging that it's not possible to be fully trauma-informed and completely safe, we try to prevent these circumstances. We recognize trauma responses as protective and don't shame them. And we work toward a calm and connected, yet authentic, environment.

How do these trauma responses show up?

FIGHT can look like a person who's irritable and grumpy. They might have misdirected anger, feelings that seemingly come out of nowhere.

They're likely the person who everyone wants to avoid. People might feel like they "walk on eggshells" around such a person. There can also be a passive-aggressive fight response: gossip, manipulation, power-grabbing, and spreading false rumors.

FLIGHT will be a person who constantly changes jobs, never feeling satisfied or content. They will have restless energy, as if they've had four cups of coffee before they even start. They could seem easily distracted, have trouble focusing, or have trouble sitting still.

FAWN might look as if a person is easy to get along with, always eager to help, and never complains—but as a "people-pleasing" trauma response, it means they're simply pretending. They never get their own needs met; instead they consider others. Society often perceives these people as desirable workers, but there's often a high price they pay with their authenticity, their dignity, and their own desires.

FREEZE shows up in this environment looking like laziness or apathy. The person is late, misses deadlines, and doesn't seem engaged when they show up. They might appear bored, staring into space, forget what's been said or their own schedule.

There are things that can be done, even if you're not a psychologist.

These are some themes to consider, which our team reflected on in designing Safer Spaces Training programs:

- *Education:* Helping people understand the trauma response that's trying to protect them, which will reduce shame and promote compassion (for self and others). This includes promoting self-awareness while also holding others accountable and gently reinforcing boundaries.
- *Skills:* It's insufficient to be aware of our own responses and reflexes, or to recognize manifestations in others. It's essential to learn practical tools to shift our nervous system, to self-reflect, and to approach our interactions.

- *Choice:* Providing students, employees, clients, or customers a range of choices, so they feel a sense of agency (control)
- *Flexibility:* Creating times outside of routine where new things are being learned, adaptations are ongoing, and establishing different patterns to ensure that the brain doesn't get stuck in traumatic responses
- *Connection:* Teaching all people how to use *ventral vagal* systems to attune to the energy in a room as well as co-regulate (tune in to each other with empathy and care)
- *Environment:* Designing spaces that suit the different ways that minds and bodies optimally interact, enhancing calm and connection. It is important to ensure that a space isn't causing inadvertent harm to marginalized communities.

Whether at work, school, or leisure—trauma responses show up along with the human. Recognizing them and learning how to prevent or manage them is key. Holding ourselves and others accountable for our actions while centering disadvantaged people. Showing up with compassion and curiosity. These are things we can all do, which will help create safer spaces everywhere.

We co-founded Safer Spaces Training to help public-facing professionals and organizations learn more. If you are interested in hiring our team, please visit SaferSpacesTraining.com. We hope to develop HR software with our modules soon.

CHAPTER 30

Communities of Practice

A *community of practice* is a group of people who share a common interest. They might meet virtually or in-person to discuss a topic or to work toward a shared objective.

In this way, the knowledge and skills become jointly owned—no one can claim to be the biggest expert. The community is the expert. They collectively create new ways of being and doing.

This is my dream for this book.

I don't want to be the keeper of knowledge—but to let it flow through. To encourage others to build on it, to make it their own.

> How do the ideas in this book fit your context?
> What works? What doesn't? Can the ideas be modified?
> In what way do the concepts help? In what way
> do they need to be shifted?

The term *community of practice* comes from education, where ideas become a "living curriculum." This concept is as old as time. Humans seek to understand how the world works and to make sense of our place here. They invented, they experimented, they created together. Within tribes, within villages, within communities.

My intention is to facilitate conversations with communities of practice around each topic in this book. On the website (through the QR code on page xviii), you'll find the video and audio recordings, as well as links into chat sites where you can share your thoughts and read the thoughts of others. Ideally, you'll add to our active resource list.

Consider these resources, as all ideas here, invitations—never expectations. The dialogue needs your voice. Your insights.

Could you host a book club and speak to your friends about these ideas? There's a book club guide (with personal information as well as suggested activities) at the QR code on page xviii.

Much of the world has been convinced that our individual desires give us meaning. That success is personal.

> What if success is a healthy community?
> What if we heal trauma to forge a more beautiful
> future for us all?

Acknowledgments

This book could not have happened without a lot of support.

My first shout-out is to my mom, Lois. She was my first editor, but also my last. Her belief in me and this work has been a powerful fuel. I love you so much.

My next thanks are to my sister, Cathy, and her family. Spending time with them brings me so much meaning and joy. Fills my bucket, as she says. I want this world to be a safe space for Kate and Ty to grow.

To my chosen family, Aishwarya Khanduja. I know you have real parents, but for me to be in your life in this way—co-mentors, co-journeying—it's incredible. You're the true butterfly, wee one.

I'm thrilled to be represented by Sam Hiyate at The Rights Factory. He's been with me as an editor on my journey writing fiction (where my style is much more literary...stay tuned.). As an agent, he shows up with tons of integrity and drive. He helped me navigate a completely foreign world. This led me to Dan Ambrosio at Hachette Go, who has been patient and flexible with my zany ideas. Alison Dalafave and Iris Bass contributed tremendously with their editing suggestions—all coordinated by Cisca Schreefel.

Huge thanks to the readers who went through the third draft and improved it greatly—with a wise lens and a keen eye for grammar. Your suggestions and resources have made this book so much better, and I'm beyond grateful to Navneet Gidda, Syma Habib, Maaria Shah, Gabriel Kwan Pok (Gabby) Yu, and Lidia Avvakoumova.

An international team worked furiously behind the scenes to make this possible. Earthly Made website design in Indonesia created the Modern Trauma online experience. (Click the QR code on page xviii if you haven't yet.) Cristina Rendon (in Mexico) did the illustrations for the website (animations) and this book. Her imagination created characters more vivid and interesting than I could have dreamed. The TRE illustration is the only one she didn't do—this was commissioned on Fiverr through Clara Tejeda Barbeito (Argentina).

To my mentors along this journey. Prof. Bob Woollard (retired UBC), for infusing life with stories and social accountability. Dr. Kate Maguire (my doctoral supervisor at Middlesex University, London), who is making grad school, and a journey into analytic autoethnography, such a pleasure. Dr. Jennifer Hatfield (retired UofC), for helping me learn about impact, intention, and partnerships. Dr. Julian Norris, for showing us how to touch the sky while keeping our toes firmly rooted in the earth. Dr. Lissa Rankin, who started as a guide in how to be a healed person while in service, but has become a dear friend (and to Zahra Ahamed who connected me, knowing exactly what I needed in my own time of trauma). And Dr. Vanessa Andreotti, who guides us to unlearn, braid, and experiment with cartographies that accept the complexities.

To my teachers in trauma. Dr. Eric Gentry helped me understand the value of attunement. To Colleen Clark, for the incredible gift of ART now in my hands. And to so many teachers in the somatic healing arts—all inspiring (credited in the Notes pages online, accessed with the QR code on page xviii). It was an honor to study with eminent pioneers in the field like Drs. Gabor Maté, Bessel van der Kolk, and Pat Ogden, who've paved the way for a new story that's emerging.

To my friends in innovation spaces, true changemakers. Jordana Armstrong, one of the most brilliant people I know. Jake Jennings, with the same learning quest and the kindest heart. Eve Blossom, and her book *Material Change*, for its wise tapestries. Dr. Frances Westley, for helping me believe that deep change was possible. Dr. Meg Wheatley, for helping me learn that the path of the Warrior can mean harnessing wisdom and kindness. Also a huge thank you to my social innovation coach, Jill Andres, who helps me dream deeper.

I've been lucky to have a large circle of humans and animals that I spend time with—Annalee Coakley, Vivian Skovsbo, and Margo Schellenberg help keep me outside where my brain heals. To Monty Ghosh, for always believing in my work and a shared passion for those placed at risk. The neighbors who make the Best Street so wonderful. My dog companion, Fife. And Wanita Lopeter, gone so long but never forgotten. To Marina, Natasha, and Svitlana, who have been sharing my home (and the dog duties) during much of the writing. *Slava Ukraini!*

To my own healing team—Fleur Yumol, Leanne Edwards, Rita Bozi, and Emma Harding—who got me through the toughest of times.

To the fellow students of all the courses and workshops I've done over the years—I still hold you in my heart. School friends like Sari Uretsky, shenanigans with Kathy Blight in med school, and Masterminds across the world. And to my fellow neurogeeks, Christine Kennedy and Vivienne Livingstone, who have an insatiable thirst for learning and send me articles to feed my brain. To the team at Global Familymed Foundation—Russel Dawe, Samina Warraich, and Besigye Innocent in Uganda—it's an honor to be doing this work with you. To everyone at the Mosaic Refugee Health Clinic (with the best docs I know), Rapid Adult Addiction Clinic, Peter Lougheed Hospital, and to those magical fairies at community health centers that deeply care about their patients (with a special shout-out to Randall Berlin). To all former students who inspire and astound me by all you've accomplished, especially those who completed the Health Equity residency when I was program director. Wow, you are amazing.

To my TikTok mutuals that teach me, sharing their wisdom and vulnerabilities. The video production team from the website is MediaPop—I met Ryan Northcott on the app. I also met Simone Saunders, one of the early team members at Safer Spaces Training. It's been such a huge blessing to meet these and so many other incredible content creators in mental health and beyond (especially Indigenous #NativeTikTok). To everyone who's supported my platform and helped me learn from theirs—it's meant so much.

To all my fellow advocates for systems change. There are friends who've bravely gone the political route, like David Swann and Jane Philpott. Others who are brilliant in medical leadership, like Katharine Smart and Alika

Lafontaine. There are local forces of resilience where I've been a member of a heartfelt coalition: environmental justice, universal health care, refugee health, decriminalization, and public health. It's incredibly hard to shift these systems but so meaningful to try.

To the energies of my father and grandmother that beat in my veins. To all my ancestors. May we each become good ancestors ourselves.

Healing, emerging from the chrysalis and flying, starts with us.

Connect with me at ChristineGibson.net—my professional page

ModernTrauma.com—and the hidden page through the QR code on page xviii

Consulting for corporations and professionals can be accessed through SaferSpacesTraining.com

Find me on TikTok at @tiktoktraumadoc, on Facebook at Christine Gibson MD, and on Twitter at @ModernTrauma. I'd love to hear from you!

Index